This Cap of White

⌁ THE STORY OF THE
MOUNDS-MIDWAY
SCHOOL OF NURSING

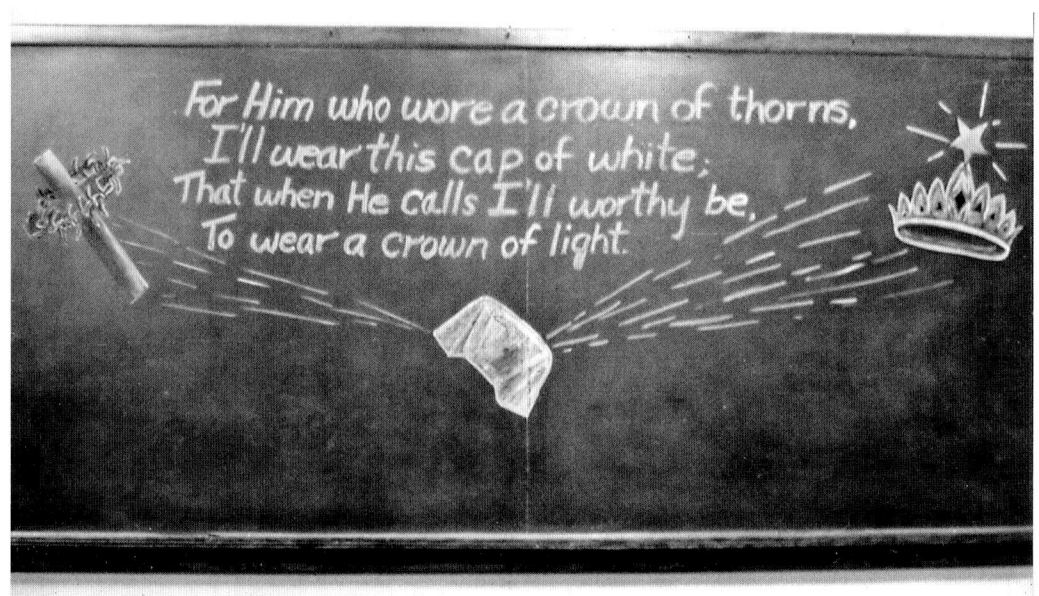

This photograph shows a chalk drawing on the front blackboard of the large classroom at Mounds Park. It was drawn by Eleanore Anderson Vogel (1950).

This Cap of White

∾ THE STORY OF THE MOUNDS-MIDWAY SCHOOL OF NURSING

Daniel John Hoisington

The Mounds-Midway Alumni Association
Edinborough Press

Saint Paul, Minnesota
2007

Copyright ©2007 by the Mounds-Midway Alumni Association, All rights reserved including the right of reproduction in whole or in part in any form.

For more information, contact:
The Mounds-Midway School Alumni Association
HealthEast Midway Campus
1700 University Avenue
Saint Paul, Minnesota 55104

Edinborough Press
P. O. Box 13790
Roseville, Minnesota 55113
1-888-251-6336
www. edinborough. com
books@edinborough. com

ISBN 1-889020-24-9

Contents

Preface 1

Acknowledgments 3

Introduction 5

Intelligent Christian Nurses 7

To Be a Nurse 37

A Sisterhood 73

My Heart, My Mind 105

The Tie That Binds 141

In Service 173

Index 179

Preface

Reading through these pages, I am reminded of so many great stories and incidents from my whirlwind days as a nursing student at Mounds-Midway School of Nursing. It's embarrassing to admit how many of those treasured stories I had forgotten over the years. But the words of this book brought me back in time and gave me the great pleasure of recalling and reflecting on my many wonderful experiences at this outstanding educational institution.

I am grateful to Adella Bennett Espelien, who captured the first 50 years of the school in her work, *A History of Mounds-Midway School of Nursing*, in 1967. In *A Cap of White* Daniel Hoisington further details those early decades, then continues with a fascinating recounting of "the rest of the story." Through research, personal interviews, letters and e-mails, he has created an intriguing compilation of 100 years of factual and anecdotal history.

Throughout these years some exceptional people have been affiliated with Mounds-Midway School of Nursing, and I am grateful that Hoisington highlighted the contributions of those extraordinary individuals. Melvin Conley (or Mel, as he now insists on being called), for example, is given well-deserved credit for his insight and perseverance in keeping our school of nursing in high regard. What an encourager, leader, and friend he was — and still is — to many former students.

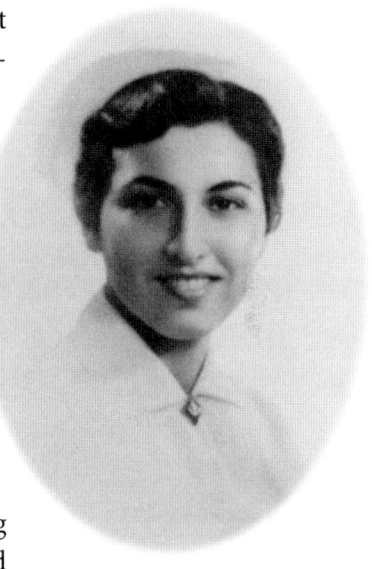

Gena Testa Schottmuller
Class of 1957

A strong spiritual foundation was the cornerstone of Mounds-Midway School of Nursing, so it was a place that many of us either began our journey of faith or built on what we believed. Hoisington underscores the unique spiritual emphasis of the school by sharing individuals' personal stories of deeply spiritual experiences in chapel or during daily prayer time in the Midway Hospital nursery. This resonated with me, as I also found those times inspiring and affirming of my faith and dependence on our living God.

Hoisington designates chapters depicting certain periods of time, so any reader with a connection to the school is sure to encounter personally relevant stories and depictions. And those items will inevitably trigger memories that are not included in the book as well. Memories, after all, are the heart of Hoisington's text. Collective memories played a key role in the development of the book, including memories of the Cadet Corp, the black stockings, the long-sleeved uniforms, and the caps with their one or two stripes. Memorable photos support some of those details as well. I love looking at the antiquated photos he includes and reading the stories about the individuals they portray.

I truly appreciate the way Hoisington has captured the essence of Mounds-Midway School of Nursing — its culture, its spiritual emphasis, and its special events, including the fun times the choir had with its various directors. Chapter One is especially intriguing in its depiction of historical figures who played a role into making our school such a successful and respected institution. How many years have we presented scholarships in the name of Kerbach-Dahlby? I knew people like this were important to the school, but after reading about them I now feel like I "know" them.

Some of the individuals quoted in *A Cap of White* I had forgotten about. Some have passed on. Yet, how moved I was emotionally to read their words and once again remember them fondly. I laughed, I cried, I remembered. Turn the page and begin reading and no doubt you will, too.

Gena Testa Schottmuller
PRESIDENT

Acknowledgments

THIS CAP OF WHITE has been a long time in the "wished-for" state as we often reminisced in the various boards and committees about the desire for a history of our school. *A History of Mounds-Midway School of Nursing, 1907—1967* by Adella Bennett Espelien, written in 1967 for the Seventy-fifth Diamond Jubilee of the school, needed to be updated to reflect the remaining fifteen years until the school closed in 1983. It sold for a dollar but many alumni were not aware of the book.

At the annual Alumni Board meeting on May 7, 2004 it was approved to go ahead with the book. Much preliminary work was done exploring other diploma school's histories and possible publishers and formats. The alumni of Swedish Hospital School of Nursing were especially helpful as their school was similar in many ways (and also closed) and they had recently completed a project to publish their second history book. *A True Nurse*. I wish to especially thank three of their members whose insights and advice were invaluable—Jesse Hanson, Edna Fordyce, and Judith Luchtenhurg Liljegren. Interestingly, Jesse's mother is a 1918 graduate of MMSN, Judy is related to Eunice Liljegren Wikstrom (1944) and Edna and Marilyne Gustafson met at Bethel, attended the University of Minnesota, and served on Nurses Christian Fellowship think tanks and both served on the editorial review board of the *Journal of Christian Nursing* since its inception. The most important Swedish Hospital alumni link is that they introduced us to the author of their book, *A True Nurse*—Daniel Hoisington—our author.

Another Swedish grad who deserved credit for preserving our history is Ruth Gustafson. Ruth served offically in the teaching and administration of our school. She was an associate director and educational coordinator at Mounds Park, 1925-1955. She came as instructress. Ida C. L. Isaacson our second director (1908-1909) was a Swedish graduate before 1899 and was their first superintendent.

Ruth Gustafson's contribution to this book is related not only to her professional one but to her collection of memorabillia about the students and graduates. Her newspaper clippings, scrapbooks, and files were priceless, as well as other items gathered by her in the first

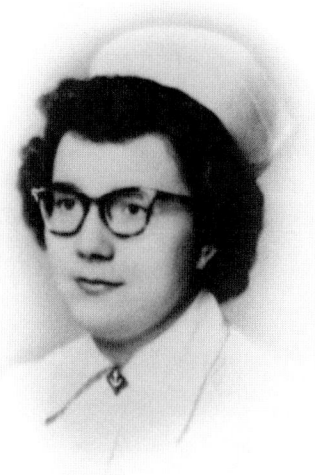

Marilyne Backlund Gustafson, Class Of 1954

museum in the lower level of Robert Earl Hall at 222 Earl Street. It started with a small closet-type room and grew to two rooms that contained files and enamel-ware equipment from the nursing arts lab.

Ruth must have corresponded with most of our missionaries. She worked tirelessly with the Anderson sisters (Char and Janice), Arlene Lick Felland, Ivy Kroll, Iona Stone Holsten, and Eleanore Anderson Vogel. When the dorm closed in 1977 the contents of the museum were packed into boxes and moved to the basement of Midway dorm. In storage the contents were damaged and records lost, but these became the basis of the current museum at Midway. Mary Jo Borglund Monson and committees used these as the foundation for the locations in 501N (the first PAR unit at Midway), 301N and now first floor museum. The original museum board deserves much credit for the museum development especially making something with dusty, damaged materials and devoting countless hours of packing and unpacking over four moves. The original surveys about various subgroups (faculty, missionaries, military and museum themes) have been very helpful.

Daniel Hoisington has led us through the process involving brainstorming, scanning photos, mailings requesting photos and articles, fund raising and interviews. Dan's perspective on societal history surrounding our clinical experiences has been refreshing. He has been patient with us as we veered "off agenda" with our reminiscing. As he poked around the present museum he delightfully informed us we have collected "good stuff" — including information about our alums and the collection of books authored by them.

The book has been an exciting adventure — especially as we get closer to completion. I want to thank the alumni board, the museum board, and especially the book committee. The photos and materials Daniel has scanned remain in the museum and for that we are very thankful. They will provide us with future opportunities to reminisce. Did I say we are fond of reminiscing?

A huge thank you to those of you who participated in scannings, and for sharing your materials and thoughts, and for your financial help. May the book not only delight us as proud graduates of MMSN but may we proclaim the praises of HIM whom we serve until we wear the crown of light, and join those who have gone before us. May we be found faithful.

Marilyne Backlund Gustafson
BOOK COMMITTEE CHAIRPERSON

Introduction

Consider me a skeptic. I have been fortunate to write history books for many organizations and small towns over the past few decades, including the story of the Swedish Hospital School of Nursing. Each place tends to be so focused on its particular history that common events appear to be unique. "Our people were hard-working," say the citizens of a farm community, when, of course, all farm people were hard-working. "We were the best," alumni will say about their school, but, from an outsider's perspective, after hearing a dozen similar claims, it is clear their experiences were shared by students at many other institutions.

And yet. Within the span of a few weeks, I interviewed a number of remarkable women — all graduates of the Mounds-Midway School of Nursing. Women like Dagmar Swanburg Brodt, who founded the Livingston University School of Nursing, and Evelyn Ellis Cohelan, who was the first dean of the George Mason University School of Nursing. and Adella Bennett Espelien, student, teacher, and director at Mounds-Midway, then longtime faculty member at the College of St. Benedict, and Beth Peterson, a 1971 graduate who began her teaching career at Mounds-Midway and continues it today at Bethel University. I picked up a devotional book by John Piper and read about the remarkable witness of Ruby Eliason. I searched the internet and stumbled on a story about the continuing contribution of the village of New Hope in Cameroon, West Africa, started by Laura Reddig.

Something special took place at the Mounds-Midway School of Nursing. Adella Bennett Espelien, who could astutely analyze the shortcomings of diploma school training, nevertheless said, "The school produced a very fine nurse. These were bright, capable people — dedicated, compassionate, very hard-working. You could not find a better or more highly-devoted group of nurses. Of course you started out with a very fine group of women."

If you begin with a carefully selected student body, then add the discipline of a typical diploma school program, you will produce quality graduates. At Mounds-Midway, there was one other element — a commitment that went beyond one's self. Many alumni recalled singing at morning chapel or convocation, "Give of your best to the Master, give of the strength of your youth." That attitude was pervasive and set a high standard for faculty, administrators, and students.

It has been a great privilege to work on this book over the past two years. What interesting people I have been able to meet — some long dead. More than two hundred graduates contributed letters, newspaper articles, or photographs for this book. Archivists at Bethel University and the Minnesota Historical Society provided welcome assistance with their collections.

The memories are sometimes faulty and the images faded. But, piece by piece, they combined to give me an understanding of the school and its legacy. Even if every story or snapshot does not appear in the following pages, all greatly increased my knowledge and made it a better book. The experience has enriched my life and encouraged me to "give of my best to the Master" as I told the story of the Mounds-Midway School of Nursing.

Daniel John Hoisington

CHAPTER ONE
Intelligent Christian Nurses

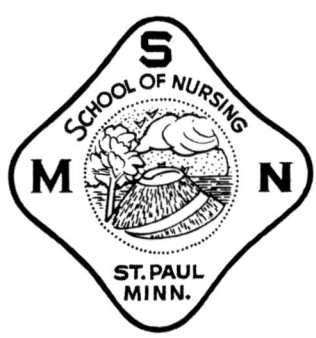

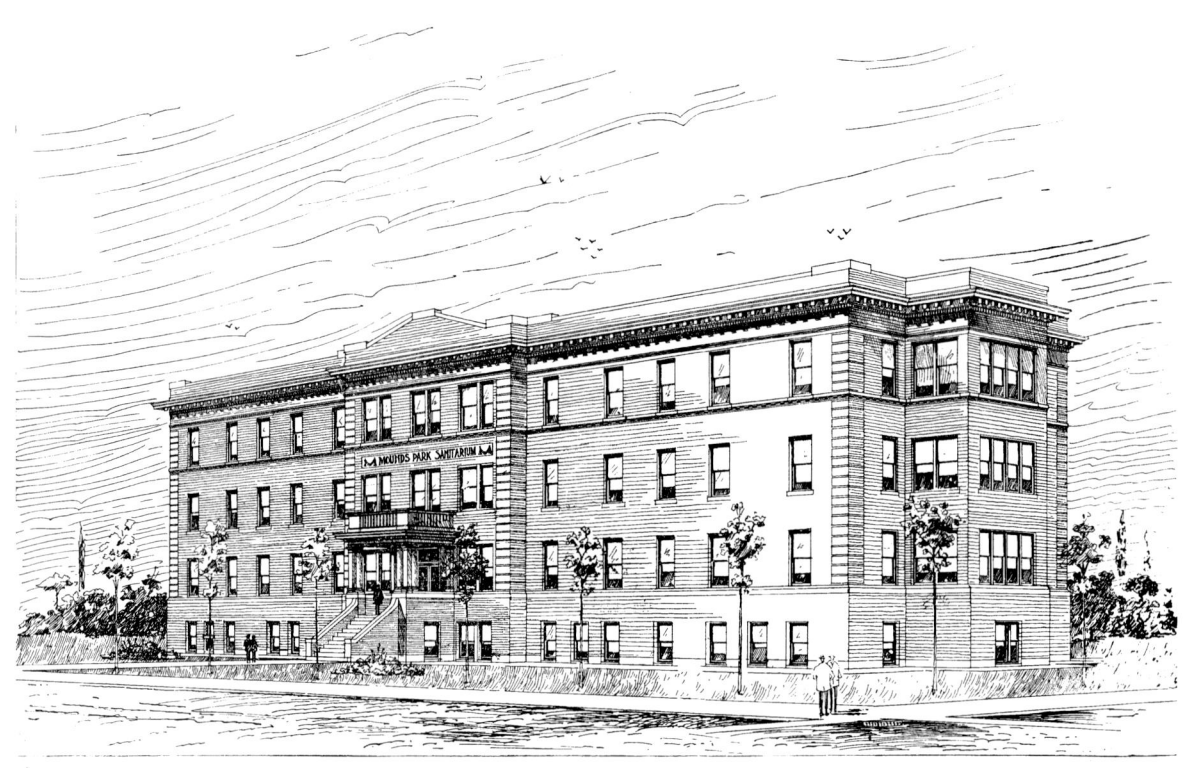

THE MOUNDS PARK SANITARIUM, ST. PAUL, MINN.

*T*HEY CALLED IT "SNOOSE Boulevard." In the years after the Civil War, thousands of Scandinavians came to Minnesota, all passing through St. Paul. At first, they moved into a neighborhood called Swede Hollow, a derelict area near the railroad tracks. By the 1890s, though, many had established themselves in business and in the community and moved up the hill toward Arlington Heights. Payne Avenue was the main street of the Swedish community in St. Paul, and according to one store owner, if he could not speak Swedish, you had no business on Payne Avenue.[1]

One of the store owners was a man named Nels Lindahl, who ran a small grocery. Born in Sweden in 1853, he came to the United States in 1881 with his wife, Sophy. Settling in the Swedish neighborhood, he became active in the First Swedish Baptist Church.

The First Swedish Baptist Church in St. Paul was established near Swede Hollow in 1873. The congregation built an imposing building on Payne Avenue in 1899. The church had a strong missionary zeal and in 1898, sent its first foreign missionary, Gerda Paulson, to Japan. After her health faltered, the church continued the work, sponsoring a member of the congregation named Mary E. Danielson, a teacher and evangelist. After a term in Japan, working in Osaka, she returned to the United States and continued her work among Japanese immigrants on the Pacific Coast.[2]

A church history called Lindahl "a promoter of good work." Indeed, he pressed the church to build an educational wing soon after the main sanctuary was completed. Backing up his words, he pledged $1000 toward the proposed addition.

But Lindahl suffered from chronic Brights disease, a sometimes painful, often fatal deterioration of the kidneys. For treatment, he traveled to Battle Creek, Michigan, to visit its nationally-famous Sanitarium founded by Dr. John Harvey Kellogg, a Seventh-Day Adventist. Kellogg came up with the word "sanitarium" to reflect his idea of a sanitary retreat for health restoration and training ("a place where people learn to stay well") rather than "sanatorium," which meant a hospital for invalids or for treatment of tuberculosis. The Sanitarium doctors advocated healthier eating, drinking fresh water, and exercising in the fresh air. Among its legacies are Kellogg's Corn Flakes.

Lindahl believed that Swedish Baptists needed just such an institution

Nels Lindahl

in Saint Paul, and turned for assistance to his physician and fellow church member, Robert Earl. Robert was born on a farm outside of Lansing, Iowa, in 1872 and might have remained there except for his father's illness. Suffering from a heart murmur, the elder Earl sold off the family farm and moved to Minneapolis when Robert was age ten. The boy eventually attended the University of Minnesota medical school and graduated in 1898. After interning at Bethesda Hospital, he opened his first office on Payne Avenue.³

Robert Earl was an ambitious man, already making a mark in his profession and his community. He was among the first local physicians to have an x-ray machine in his office, and among the first owners of an automobile in St. Paul, always, said his brother, "insisting not only on good appearance but speed." Active in civic affairs, he was appointed in 1905 to a special three-person commission charged with finding a location for a children's hospital managed by his friend, Arthur Gillette. As a member of the St. Paul Parks Commission, he suggested a site near Lake Phalen, where the city was rapidly acquiring land — soon the location of the Gillette Children's Hospital.⁴

He had another vision. At medical school, he had come under the tutelage of Dr. C. Eugene Riggs, Professor of Mental and Nervous Diseases. Riggs was a pioneer in the field of nervous and mental diseases and wanted a general hospital where "the true relation of neurology to disease" was understood. Earl later said that the choice

Dr. Robert O. Earl was one of the key founders of the Mounds Park Sanitarium.

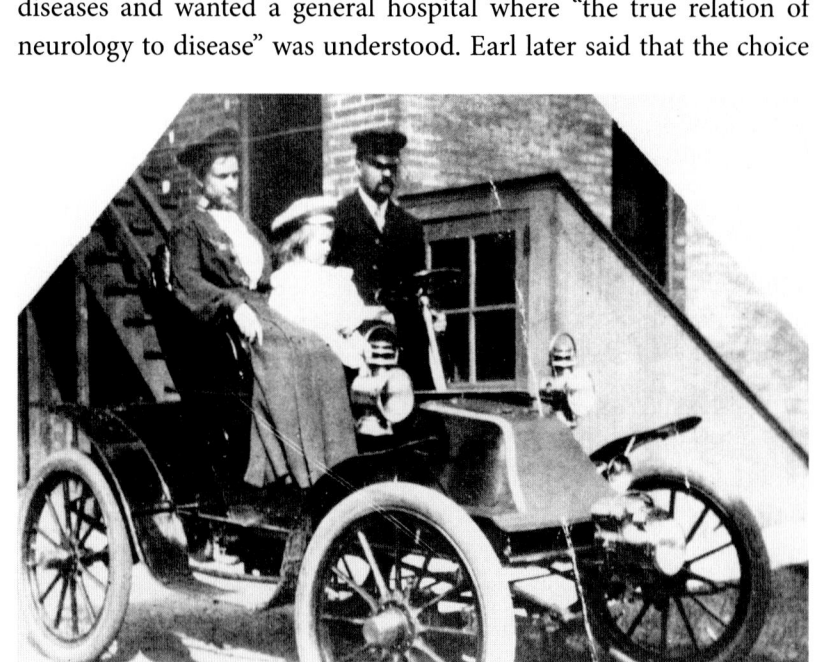

Dr. Earl owned one of the first automobiles in Saint Paul. He is pictured here with his wife and daughter around 1905.
MINNESOTA HISTORICAL SOCIETY

to go ahead with a new hospital was a difficult decision because the field was relatively new, and was not well understood or even accepted among conservative Christians.[5]

So, when approached with the idea of a new hospital, Earl heartily agreed. The two organized a meeting at Lindahl's home on Payne Avenue on November 9, 1904, attended by church members Olof Swenson, a local builder, and Carl P. Dahlby, a plumbing contractor. These men organized the Mounds Park Sanitarium Association in early 1905. The purpose of the association was:

> To found and maintain in the city of Saint Paul, Minnesota, a sanitarium or hospital, wherein to care for the bodily ills of the sick, wounded, feeble and afflicted, and to provide attention, care, and nursing, and the services of intelligent physicians and surgeons, to aid in the restoration of such persons to health and strength, and thereby do deeds of Christian charity and incident thereto, to minister in the name of Christ to their spiritual needs and welfare.[6]

The first board of directors included Dr. Robert Earl, president, as well as Nels Lindahl, Pastor Larson, Olof Swenson, and Dr. Arvid Gordh, the president of Bethel Academy.

The church was fortunate, within a few months, to come under the leadership of the man named Magnus Larson. Pastor Larson seized on the idea, and throughout the summer of 1906, he traveled to Swedish Baptist churches in the upper Midwest, accompanied by a quartet from the church, to raise money for the new hospital.[7]

Given the inspiration of the Battle Creek Sanitarium, with its emphasis on a healthy environment, it is not surprising that the Association insisted on a proper location. They acquired property in an area known as the Indian Mounds Park, high on a bluff overlooking the Mississippi River. The association explained the choice:

> Since patients come from long distances and from all directions, it is necessary that the hospital be located in a large railroad center, and within a short distance from the depot, so as not to exhaust the sick and feeble patient by a long, tedious, and expensive ride in an ambulance or carriage. The location should also have good streetcar service, together with all the conveniences of the city, such as city water, sewer, gas, and electricity for light and power. It

C. Eugene Riggs, a pioneer in the field of neurosurgery, taught Robert Earl at the University of Minnesota. He served on the staff at Mounds Park Sanitarium for many years.

The first board of directors included Dr. Robert Earl, Nels Lindahl, Pastor Magnus Larson from the First Swedish Baptist Church, Dr. Arvid Gordh, president of Bethel Academy, and Olof Swenson, a building contractor.

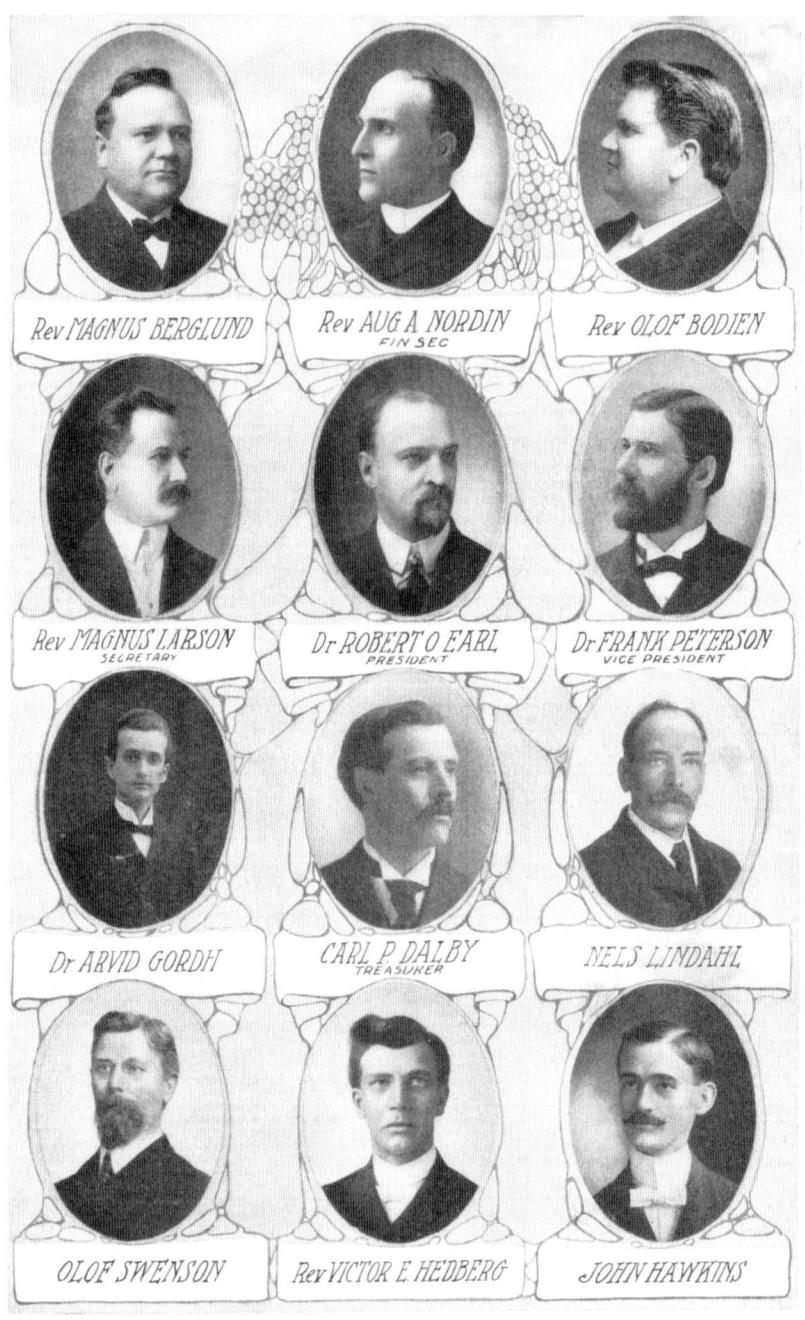

is also of great importance that the institution should be built in a healthful community, out of the way of the noise, dust, and smoke of the center of a busy city, where ample grounds for outdoor recreation can be secured, and pure, fresh air is abundant.

Ground was broken in the spring of 1906.

Lindahl would not see the official opening of the hospital. In September 1906, he finally succumbed to his illness with Dr. Earl at his bedside. Magnus Larson moved on as well. In 1908 he suffered a serious accident returning from a funeral. Taken to the new Mounds Park Sanitarium for emergency surgery, he remained there for three months, eventually resigning to become the financial secretary of Bethel Academy.

With the approaching opening of the hospital, the Association began a drumbeat of promotion, claiming the following advantages:

- A modern fireproof general hospital for the treatment of all non-contagious diseases. Fully equipped laboratories for the diagnosis of disease.
- Modern operating and sterilizing rooms for equipment.
- Special facilities for the care and treatment of nervous disease.
- Completely equipped for the treatment of disease by hydro-therapy, electro-therapy, thermo-therapy, massage, Swedish movements, etc.
- Rates no higher than at other hospitals.

A School of Nursing

All that remain was to staff the hospital. For this, the association took what had become the traditional course and opened the Mounds Park Sanitarium School of Nursing with the stated purpose:

> The chief objects of our Association are, so far as our means will permit: to assist in the restoration to health and strength of the sick poor who are unable to pay; the spreading of the Gospel of Christ; the training of intelligent Christian nurses, who will be capable of going out into the world and administering to the physical and spiritual welfare of suffering humanity.[8]

Nursing in Minnesota was undergoing a revolution in 1907. The profession was relatively new, as Dr. Riggs remembered: "In 1881 there

Ground-breaking ceremonies for the Mounds Park Sanitarium.
MINNESOTA HISTORICAL SOCIETY

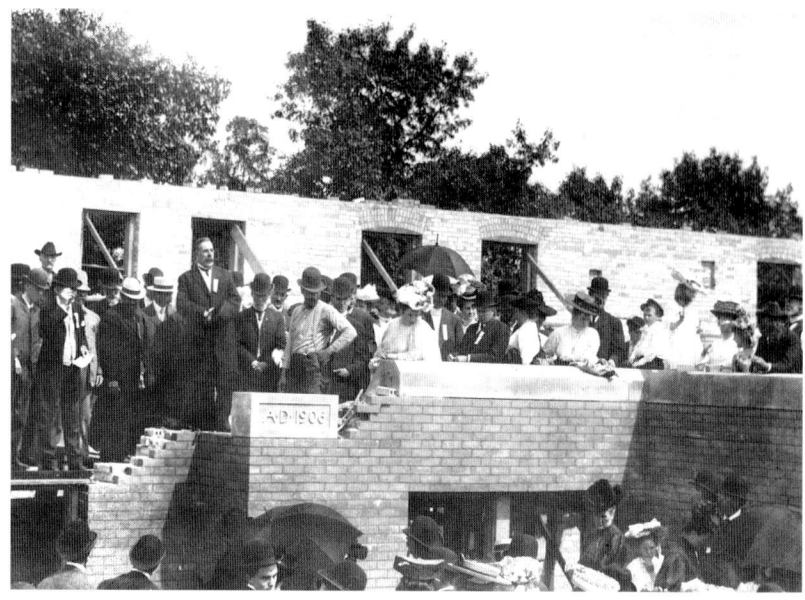

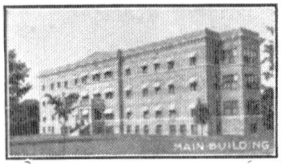

Advertisement in a Swedish language newspaper published in Chicago, 1912.

was no such thing as a trained nurse in the state of Minnesota. I am informed that St. Paul possessed one five years later and that patients vied with one another for her services."

Between 1892 and 1905, more than a dozen nursing schools opened in the Twin Cities. The system was simple. Hospitals established schools of nursing to staff the wards. In return for the long hours of work, the students received training, board, lodging, two weeks vacation, and free basic health care.[9]

As programs proliferated throughout the United States, nurses began to take it into their own hands to raise the standards of the largely unregulated training schools. One step was to establish standards to determine who qualified as a professional. In 1898, the first nurses' registry in the United States was established by the Ramsey County Graduate Nurses Association. Seven years later, Twin Cities nurses joined together to create the Minnesota State Graduate Nurses Association, whose purpose was to conduct "a society for social enjoyment and the advancement of the nursing profession in the state of Minnesota and elsewhere." Within two years they had achieved their immediate goal, which was to require state registration and licensing of nurses by a state board of examiners. Only then could they use the precious initials, R.N., next to their name.

From the beginning, Dr. Earl and Dr. Riggs set high standards for the training school, hiring Caroline Monk as the first superintendent.

The First Class

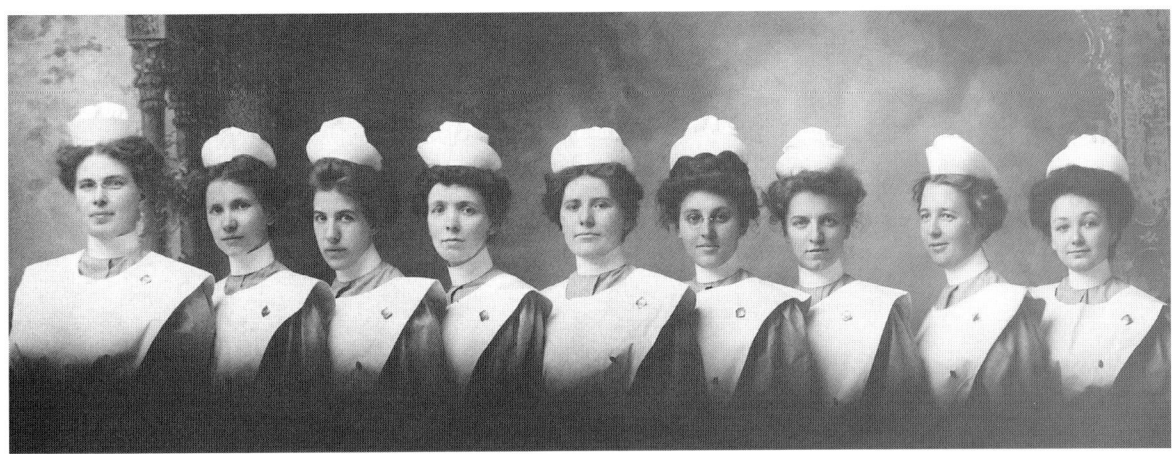

The Class of 1909. Left to right: Selma Bergh, Rose Bergstrom, Hattie Fredine, Augusta Martinson, Marie Hoppe, Edith Rydeen, Elizabeth Smith, Jennie Teberg, Jennie Warner, Stephanie Werner

Right: Mounds Park Sanitarium staff and students, circa 1909.

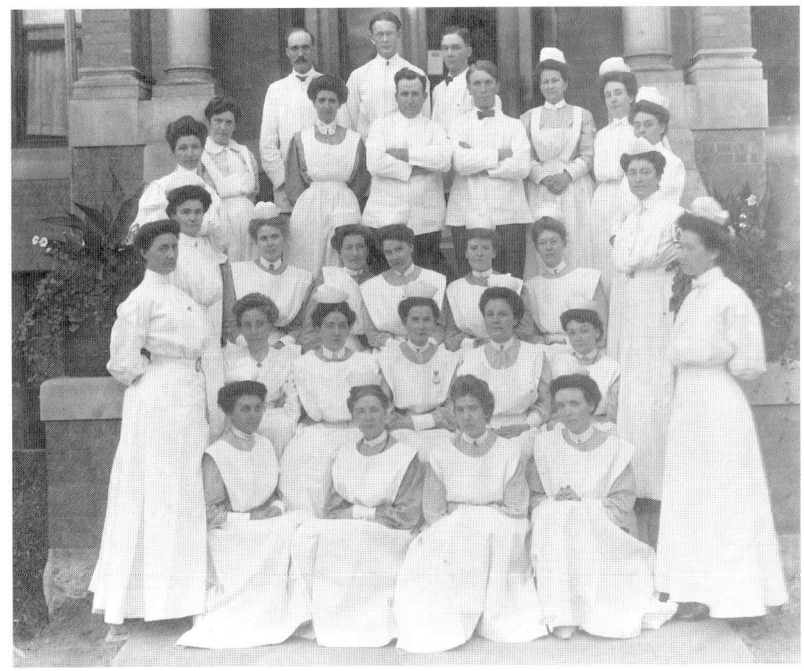

While many of the details of her life remain obscure, we know that Monk came from Canada in the 1890s and worked for several years at St. Luke's Hospital, which had an insanity ward run under supervision of a woman superintendent that Riggs singled out for praise.[10]

The hospital association turned to Ida Isaacson to develop the first curriculum. Isaacson was a graduate of the Augustana Hospital School of Nursing in Chicago and had come north to Minnesota in 1897 to serve as the first superintendent of the Swedish Hospital School of Nursing. Already widely respected in the Twin Cities for her professional skill and moral character, she was, as one former student said, "very dignified. Miss Isaacson demanded respect." Although she would leave the school in a few years and return to direct at Swedish Hospital, she created a core curriculum that remained in place until the 1920s. She left another long-term legacy — the powder blue color of the student dress.[11]

On January 7, 1907, Selma Bergh of Kerkoven, Minnesota, and Jenny Teberg, of Litchfield, Minnesota, arrived at the front door of the new hospital. Teberg might have been typical of the early applicant — twenty-one, single, spoke Swedish as a second language, with one year of high school. After being assigned a room in the annex and donning their crisp, new uniforms, they met Caroline Monk. Jenny Teberg recalled the encounter: "We were timid and somewhat awe-stricken by what seemed to be a severe and untouchable person. However, we soon found that under this starched uniform was a very kind and warm-hearted woman."[12]

The first patient — Mrs. Florence Thorp from Minnetonka — entered the hospital that same morning. By evening of that first day, the two new student nurses had been assigned three patients in the general wards.

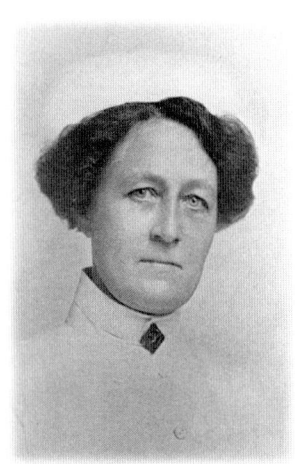

Ida Isaacson helped to develop the first curriculum and served as director of the School of Nursing for one year.

> Since there was no one to go on night duty, Miss Bergh was asked to spend the night on a cot in a patient's room. This patient was quite ill. I was asked to spend the night on a cot in the corridor near the bell box (we had bells and not lights to summon a nurse fifty years ago) so that I could wait on the two other patients on general, should they need attention. I slept all night, and so did the patients. Everything was new and so different from anything we had experienced before that we felt as though we had been dropped into a new world.

The First Student

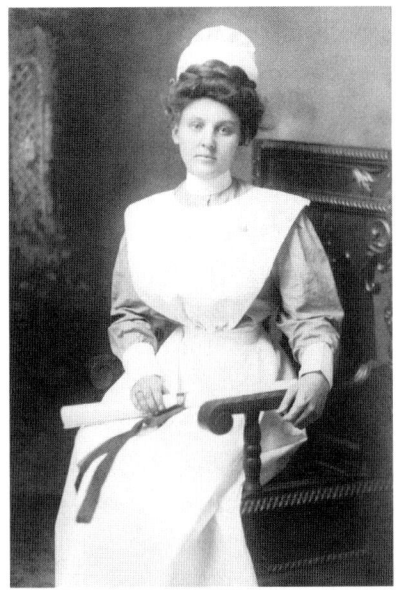

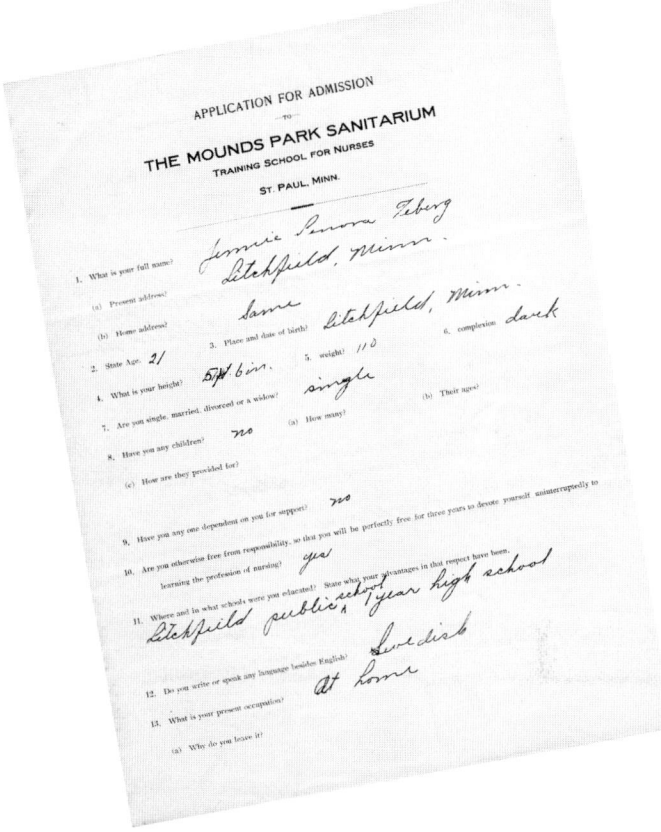

Jennie Teberg (later Paquette) was the first student to enroll in the school of nursing. Above: Teberg's application form. Left: Ledger page from 1909, showing Teberg's studies.

The next day, Jennie Warner, another new student, arrived and was quickly assigned night duty on the second floor. This first class eventually grew to ten "probies" — officially accepted as students on March 7, 1907.[13]

If the purpose of the Association was to train "intelligent Christian nurses," there was no clear path as to how to accomplish the goal. As one graduate recalled, "Nurses training was just beginning to come into its own." The superintendents, except for Caroline Monk and Ida Isaacson, were barely removed from student days. Ruth Martin, for example, became director in 1910 only six months after graduation, following a brief post graduate course at the nationally-respected Bellevue Hospital in New York. After five years as Superintendent of Nurses at Mounds, she left for two years, but returned in 1919 as hospital manager. Margaret Fortune, who followed Miss Martin in 1915, had graduated from Brandon General Hospital in Manitoba in 1913.[14]

The widely-accepted view was that the training of nurses was more an apprenticeship than a college education. Applicants were accepted for a probationary period — two months in length during the school's first decade — so that the hospital could assess their aptitude, stamina, and moral character. They were required only to have finished eighth grade — a standard that only changed in the 1920s. In the early years, the belief was that "many self-educated young women are really excellent students." For example, Mary Danielson, later director for more than thirty years, had a single year of high school.

An early catalogue explained that, "Twenty-three to twenty-five is the ideal because by that time any physical defect will have developed, the applicant will have the benefit of other experiences in life, will have more firmly established character, and will realize more fully the broad significance of this calling." Again, as an example, Mary Danielson was twenty-six when she completed the program.

Sound moral character was a prerequisite. Stephanie Werner Swenamson, one of the first students, recalled, "All the girls were so nice, brought up in good homes, with a healthy respect for religion." In those early years, most applicants were Scandinavian and Protestant. A 1923 survey of church preferences showed that, among 178 graduates, seventy-four were Baptists, followed by forty-two Lutherans. Somewhat surprisingly, nine responding graduates were Catholic.[15]

The basic requirement, though, was that they be able to work. Marriage, then, was out of the question, since family obligations would

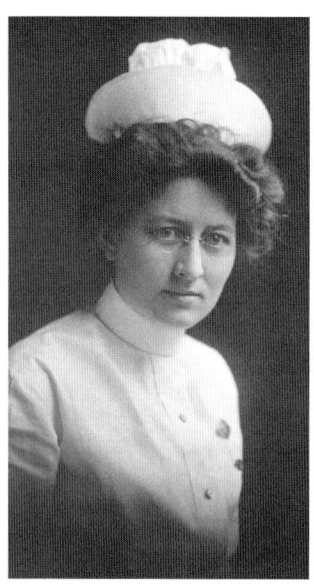

Ruth Martin graduated from Mounds in 1910, then stepped into the director's position. She held the post until 1915, then worked as a nurse during World War I. She returned for two years, eventually leaving to become supervisor of the Red Wing General Hospital.

only interfere with the long hours. When candidates were accepted, the hospital expected them to "respond promptly and to bring with them garments and personal articles specified on [the] list furnished." These included:

> 1. Three gingham dresses like sample, made with plain waist, long sleeves, gored skirt with five-inch hem, skirt not more than nine inches from the floor, gingham to be shrunk before being made up. Uniform collars may be purchased at the school.
> 2. Eight aprons and bibs and straps of loosely woven sheeting two yards wide made the length of the skirt, bottom hem five inches wide, gathered at the top of a band two inches wide.
> 3. Four sets of plain underclothing distinctly marked with full name on neck or waistbands. Warm underwear and outing flannel nightgowns for cold weather.
> 4. Two colored petticoats of wash material.
> 5. Two pair of comfortable shoes with broad toes and rubber heels (cantilevers or modified ground grippers are advised).
> 6. Bathrobe and slippers of modest color.
> 7. Sweater.
> 8. Raincoat, rubbers, umbrella.
> 9. Two bags one yard square for laundry,
> 10. Watch with second hand; fountain pen; pair of blunt-edge scissors.
> Each probationer should bring $15 to pay for required books. [16]

The training of a nurse was grounded in experience under the supervision of graduate nurses and physicians, interspersed with lectures and demonstrations. Dr. George Earl explained the rationale behind the teaching method:

> With work that is so important as dealing with the human body, and so serious as that connected with illness, it is necessary to have most careful supervision and consequently during the training years the nurse can not be given the same leeway that she could if she were studying some other profession that did not involve life. In other professions she could be left more to her own resources and learn by experience, rather than by precept and example. Those responsible for the training of student nurses must first

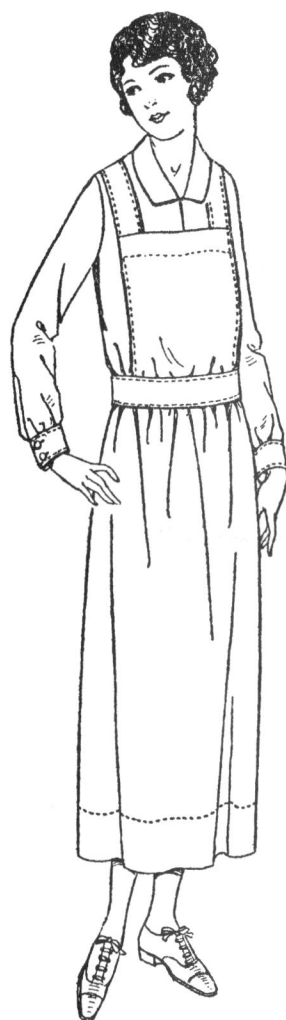

Early Probationers' dress and apron

think of the human lives under their care, but at the same time the training throughout the course should be such that individual initiative should be encouraged.[17]

The earliest training course required that the student nurse work long hours. Students began shortly after they were admitted to the school, no matter what time of year. One graduate, class of 1912, remembered, "Our day began at 7 a.m. and ended at 7 p.m. with two hours off each day, a half day off each week, and the precious four hours off on Sundays. There were no graduate nurses on each floor, no graduate night supervisors, or surgical supervisors in those days. We all had our turn in these capacities as part of our training." Practical experience included "rotations" in the various departments, somewhat weighted toward those with the heaviest patient load.

Preliminary Period	2 months
Medical Patients	10 months
Surgical Patients	6 months
Nervous and mental Patients	3 months
Obstetric Patients	4 months
Pediatric Patients	1 month
Diet Kitchen	3 months
Operating Room	3 months
Dressing Room	1 month
Pharmacy	2 weeks
Drug Room	2 weeks
Vacation	2 months
Total	36 months[18]

Classes were taught by staff physicians or nurses, except for a required Bible Studies class. The school also brought in a masseuse to instruct the students and work with patients. Viola Olson Paul (1915) wrote, "Remember our classes in massage with Mrs. Olson? I can see her yet in my memory, tripping along the halls so straight and sprightly. The patients all loved these massages given with her capable hands and we loved her as a teacher." The male masseur, she recalled, smelled of cocoa butter.

In the first years, classes included:

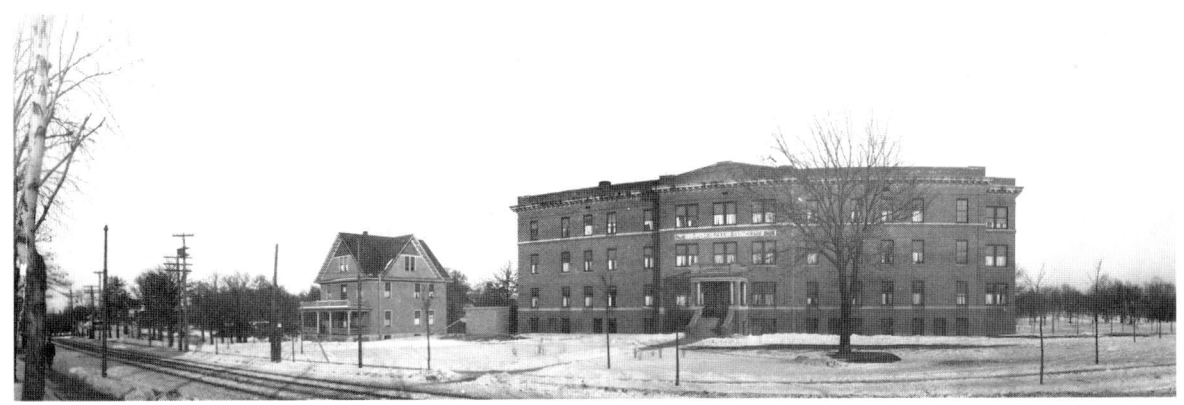

Mounds Park Sanitarium, circa 1915
MINNESOTA HISTORICAL SOCIETY

Right: The hospital grounds, shown here in 1918, had tennis and croquet courts.

Below: Mounds Park Sanitarium around 1915. The beautiful surroundings of the hospital was considered of great importance for mental health.

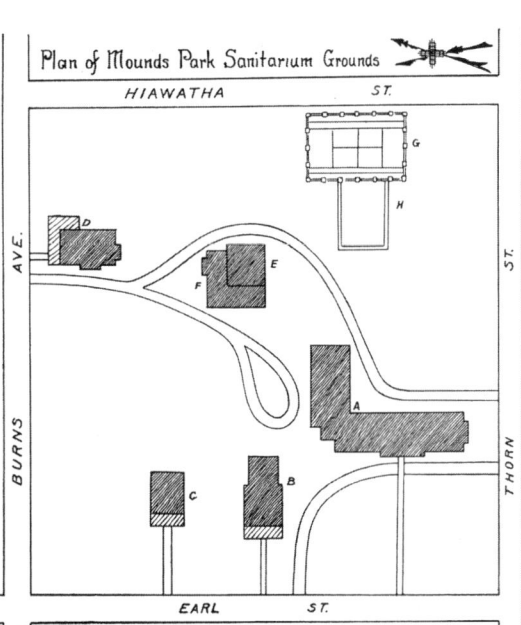

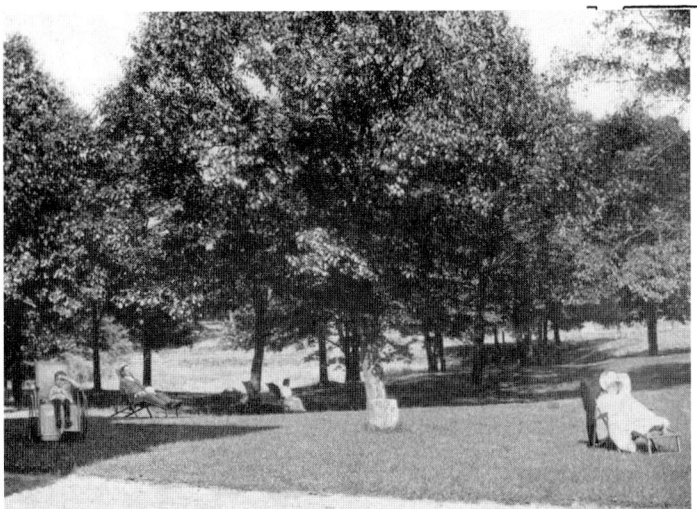

Chapter One 21

SUBJECT	HOURS TAUGHT	TEACHER
Eye, Ear, Nose, and Throat	6	Dr. Little
Contagious Diseases	10	Dr. Burns
Materia Medics	15	Ida C. L. Isaacson
Nursing Ethics	10	Miss Isaacson
Nursing Practice	30	Miss Monk
Medical Diseases	30	Dr. Dahleen
Hydroelectro therapy	2	Dr. Ball
Neuropsychiatry	12	Dr. Riggs
Bible Studies	10	Rev. Sohlquist
Anatomy and Physiology	30	Dr. Robert Earl
Blood and Urinalysis	6	Dr. Hammes
Pediatrics	10	Dr. George Earl
Dietetics	15	Miss Tanner
Surgical Nursing	10	Mrs. Marvis
Obstetrics	10	Dr. McLaren
Dermatology	10	Dr. Cook
Drugs and Solutions	15	Miss Isaacson
Medical Legal Course	1	Mr. Bernquist
Bacteriology	10	Dr. George Earl
TOTAL	242 hours	

This curriculum conformed to the best practices of the day and the early hospital staff was well-respected. Unlike many other schools, Mounds Park received accreditation almost at once.

Life as a Student Nurse

The life of a student nurse began with the arrival at Mounds Park Hospital. Viola Olson Paul (1915) wittily recalled her introduction to the school by the senior class.

> The probies huddled on the piazza of the Nurses' Home on that last, unforgettable day of August. An attempt to describe the mingled emotions of the bevy of girls gathered would exceed my abilities. Nevertheless, there they sat, when a sudden silly burst of laughter came from the doorway, and what should arrest the eyes of the probationers but a flash of scarlet shoes — on the feet of a Senior! I must confess that upon this point we experienced a slight release of tension; surely the Senior nurses must be people of like passions such as we!

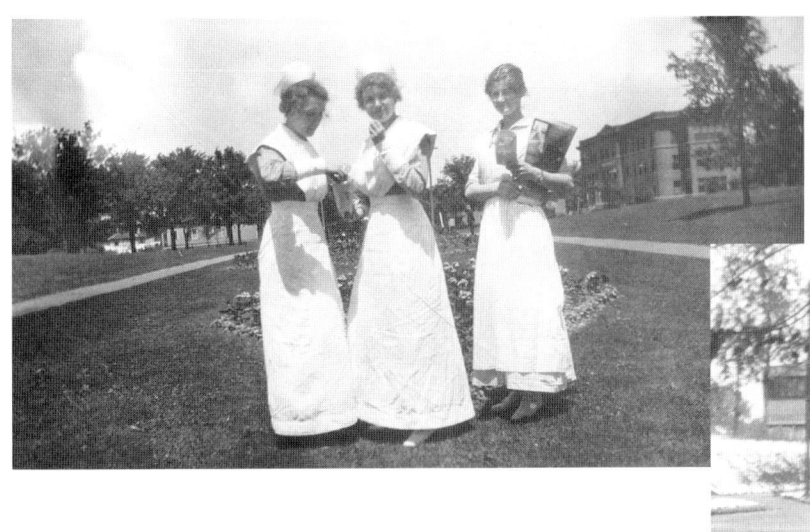

Student life in the early years. Above: The photograph, taken in October 1915, does not identify the students. Right: Leona Peterson (1927) and an unidentified fellow student enjoy a candy bar on the street outside Mounds Park. Below: "As Others See Us" from a school publication in 1922.

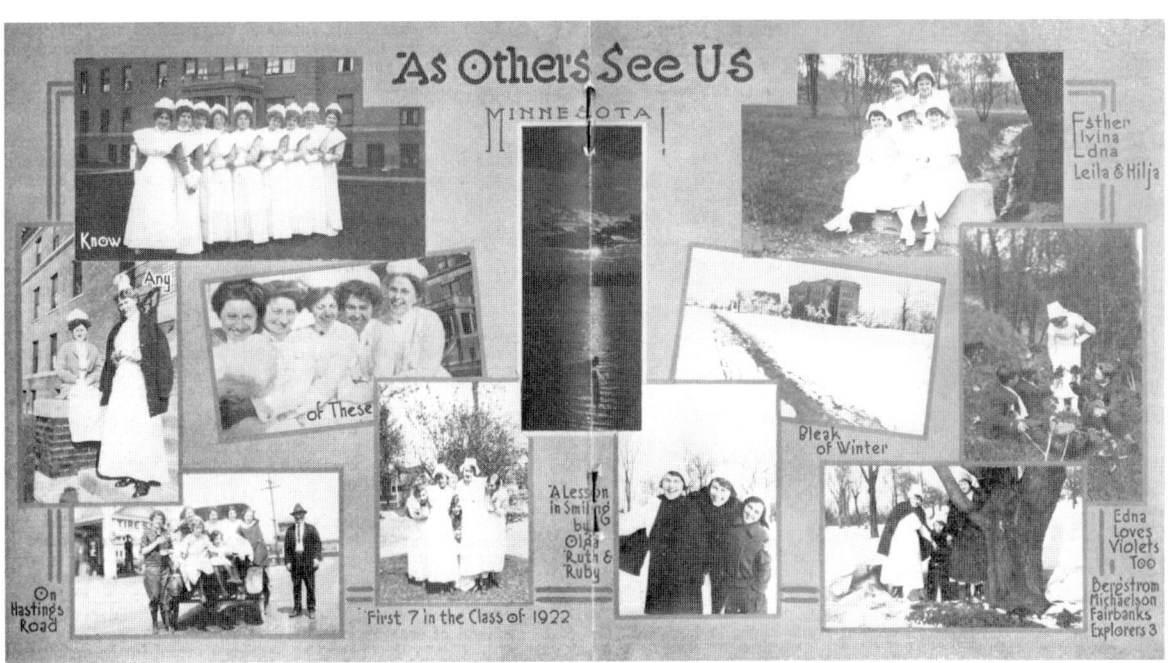

Chapter One 23

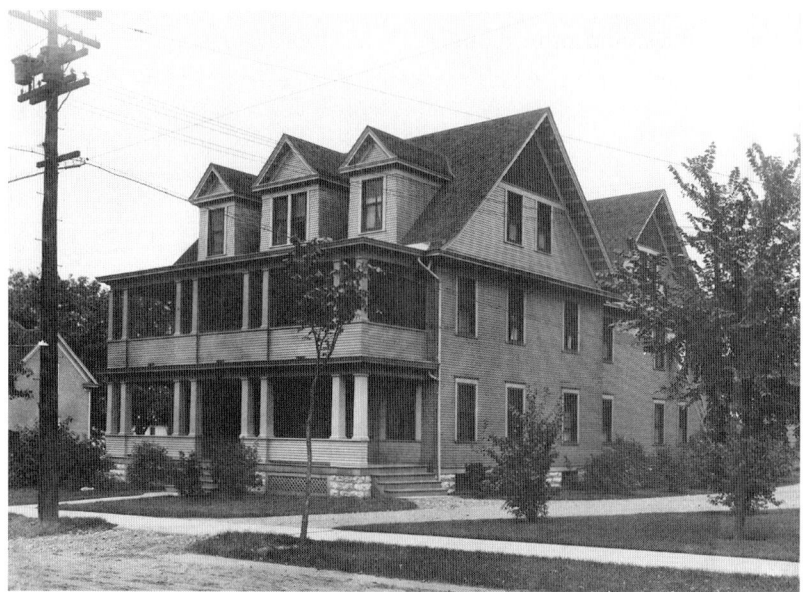

A new dorm was built in 1921 at 222 Earl Street.

With tongue in cheek, she continued:

> Yet our awe continued and increased from day to day. Were not the Seniors those who knew positively and unwaveringly every joint and muscle attachment in the human body? Was it not they who administered enemas without a quiver and charted a postmortem without the blinking of an eyelash?

"Ours was a home-like atmosphere," wrote Stephanie Werner Swenamson (1909). Students lived on the third floor of the hospital. "I remember," Swenamson continued, "the long hours we had at the hospital, but also the grand meals, our very nice rooms, and ten o'clock coffee which helped immeasurably to shorten the long, hard day." Within a few years, students moved into a small house called Hiawatha Home. With growing enrollment, in 1921, the school built a three-story house at 222 Earl Street. Its upper floors had dorm rooms, while the ground floor had a lecture room, nursing arts laboratory, and a dietetic laboratory. The library was on the first floor.

Student days were not simply long hours of work.

Remarking on the celebration of Christmas, 1922, a student wrote, "Christmas was a very merry season here. The parlor was made very inviting by the big Christmas tree and the fireplace. Eats were to be found wherever we went." Indeed, the hard-working young women showed a keen appreciation for food and holidays were routinely celebrated with cakes, cookies, and other goodies. "The popular saying," shared one student, "seems to be 'when do we eat? or 'why don't my clothes fit me anymore?'" Even classes could prove a useful source. One student recalled, "Our dietetics class tried ever so hard to display all the knowledge and skill we acquired in our classes by dividing into two sections and giving dinners for ourselves and guests. Soup was not spilled, the table was not upset and the guests did not leave before the dinners were over, so all in all we feel that we did very well."

Hazel Ahlstrom Addington (1918) gave a rare glimpse of life as a student nurse when she reminisced about the "old days" in 1928. She wrote:

> There is not a great deal of difference in nurses now and then. Night nurses still must take all the blame for things done and undone, underclassmen still rebel at senior authority. Someone is always having a late "per" withheld, but then there are still the parties and picnics and a variety of good times that do not take all the joy out of life.

There was always a time for laughter. Two students, Anna Carlson Larson and Pearl Jackson Myhre (both 1918) recalled one patient, a Rev. Winger, who suffered from insomnia. Larson wrote, "He would walk up and down the corridor — scuff, scuff, scuff — all night long." Apparently, it was memorable thirty years later, when they wrote their stories, because Mary Danielson made ghostly sounds from the operating room and "scared [the Reverend] out of a year's growth."

Almost as soon as the first graduates stepped out the door, they organized the Mounds Park Hospital Alumnae Association in 1909 with Rose Bergstrom (1909) as its first president. Dues were $1 per year, with all graduates of the school eligible to join. The purposes of the Mounds Park Alumnae Association were:

> 1. For mutual help and improvement in professional work and for promotion of good fellowship among graduates of this school.
> 2. For the advancement of interest in the Mounds Park Sanitarium School of Nursing.

3. To work for the promotion of professional and educational advancement of nursing.

4. To cooperate with the Fourth District Nurses Association, the Minnesota State Registered Nurses Association, and the American Nurses Association.

The Association carried on annual events, such as a tea, and maintained a list of graduates in order to track their postgraduate activities. They also joined in the fun. In April 1924, they hosted the seniors at a "Hard Times" party, which proved to be an initiation rite for the soon-to-be graduates. After enduring "all the abuse and torture that the heartless Alumnae had planned for them," one senior wrote: "We surely appreciate the [hazing] that they gave us because we can now sympathize with our patients."

Not for Ourselves

The Class of 1912's class motto was "Not for Ourselves" and the statement neatly expresses the school's mission to send its students "out into the world." From its earliest days, its graduates built a remarkable record of service.

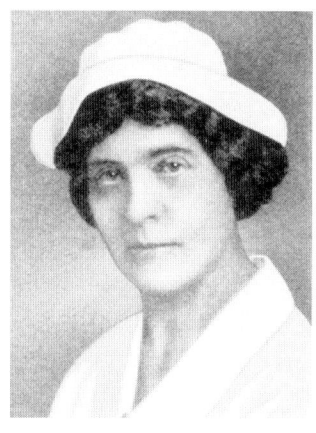

Esther Hokanson (1911) was the first of many graduates who served on the mission field.

Among the graduates of the class of 1911 was Esther Hokanson (1911). She had served as a missionary before coming to Mounds and then, after her training, returned to become superintendent of nurses in the Union Hospital in Huchow, China. In subsequent years, her work was multiplied many times over. She became director of a small school of twenty nurses and wrote text books on anatomy and personal hygiene in English and Chinese used throughout that country. "The school was truly a door through which I entered a larger life and more satisfying service," she later wrote. "Never have I found higher ideals, a more Christian atmosphere, or unselfish service than I found in the days of my training at Mounds Park."[19]

Other graduates headed to the mission field as well. Rosalie Olson (1917) was sent by the Home Mission Board of the Baptist Church to the Latin Quarter of New York City, moving on to Mexico in 1924. Edna Michaelson Anderson (1923) was sent to Assam, India. Ruth Johnson Berg (1925) also headed to Assam, then Burma, with her husband. Margaret Rinell Jewett (1922) worked as a floor supervisor at a hospital in Beijing under the auspices of the American Baptist Convention.

Following President Wilson's call to war in April 1917, women sought to find a role within the national effort. Almost at once the call went

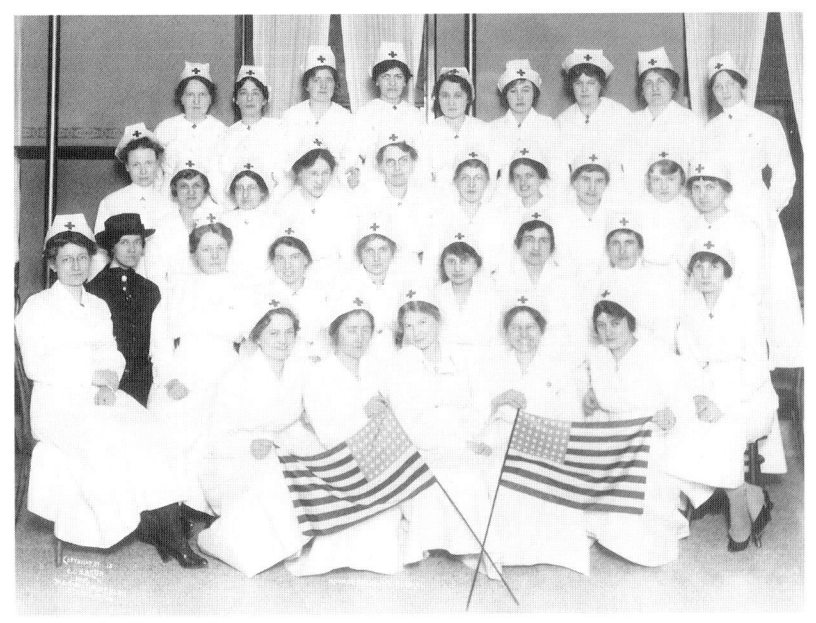
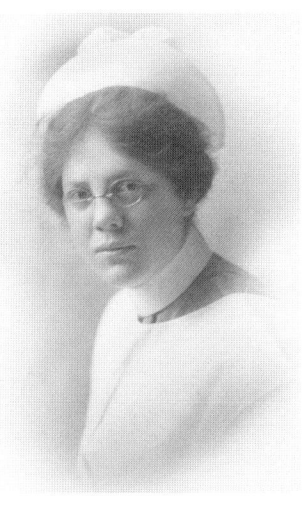

Above: These Mounds Park School of Nursing graduates joined the Red Cross during World War I. Below: In 1918, the student nurses and instructors show their support for the war effort.

Anna Dahlby (1916) volunteered as a nurse during the war and died while in service.

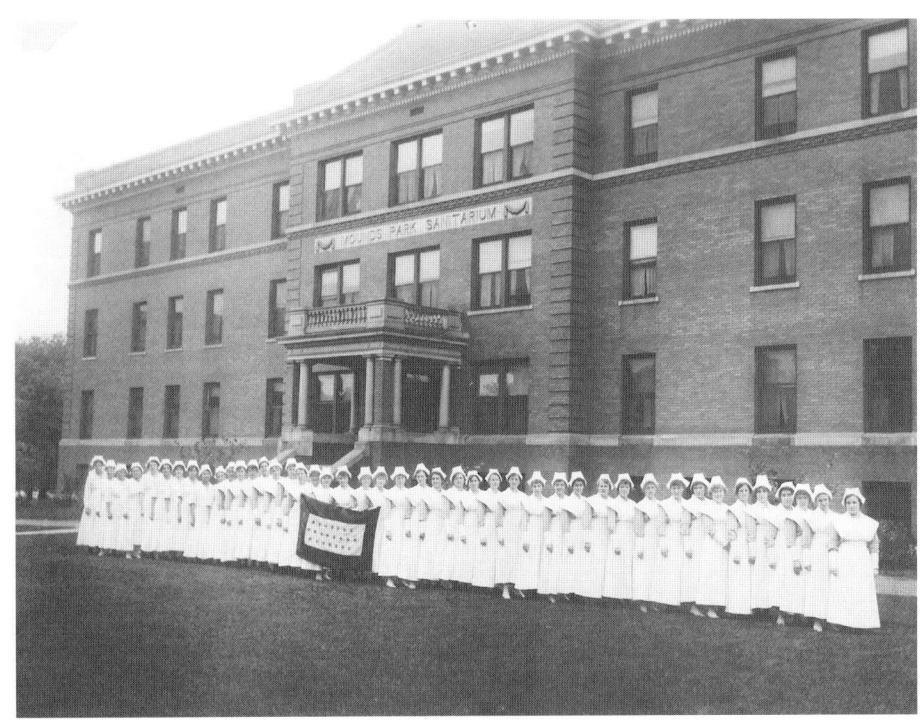

Chapter One 27

out for nurses, to be handled under the auspices of the American Red Cross. By war's end, some twenty-three thousand women had seen service as nurses. This number including several from the Mounds Park Hospital School of Nursing—seven of nine graduates from the class of 1917 served during World War I. Many entered the Navy and were assigned to the massive Great Lakes Naval Training Station north of Chicago, although Helen Drinane joined the Army Nurse Corps and served in France.

Two graduates lost their lives. Esther Kirbach (1912) enlisted in the Red Cross, and was sent to northern Minnesota to care for forest fighters. While there, Esther came down with influenza, one more victim of the worldwide pandemic. Within a few months, Anna Dahlby (1916), daughter of one of the hospital's founders, succumbed to the same disease at a military camp in Newport News, Virginia. To remember their sacrifice, the school raised money to establish the Kirbach-Dahlby Scholarship. Given to the member of the graduating class with the highest academic standing, its purpose was to encourage further studies. Karen Ryden received the first award in 1928, although she did not use the money. Almyra Eastlund won the scholarship in 1931 and used the funds to take a nursing education course at Western Reserve, subsequently heading a school of nursing in Assam, India. Another top-ranked student, Violet Nelson, received the award in 1936, but turned down the money, intent on educating a new generation of nurses rather than pursing graduate studies.

These war years brought a dramatic change to the profession. On top of the drive to win the war, the influenza epidemic of 1918 and the high rates of maternal and infant death led to major developments in local public health law. By the time the pandemic was finally over in Minnesota at the end of 1920, more than 75,000 people had been stricken, leaving nearly 12,000 dead. Rather than retrench at war's end, the Red Cross began a new Minnesota program aimed at prevention and education through the employment of nurses in public health.

Isabel Maitland Stewart, longtime chair of the Curriculum Committee of the National League of Nurses, wrote in 1921:

> Probably the greatest contribution of the war experience to nursing lies in the fact that the whole system of nursing education was shaken for a little while out of its well-worn ruts and brought out of its comparative seclusion into the light of public discussion and criticism. When so many lives hung on the supply of nurses, people

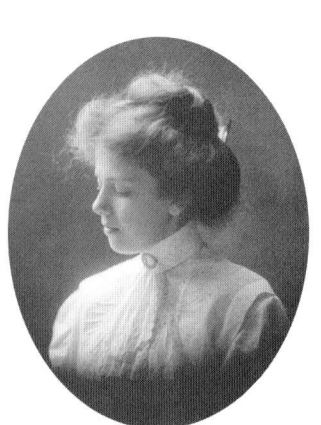

Esther Kirbach (1912), another volunteer, died while caring for forest fighters in northern Minnesota.

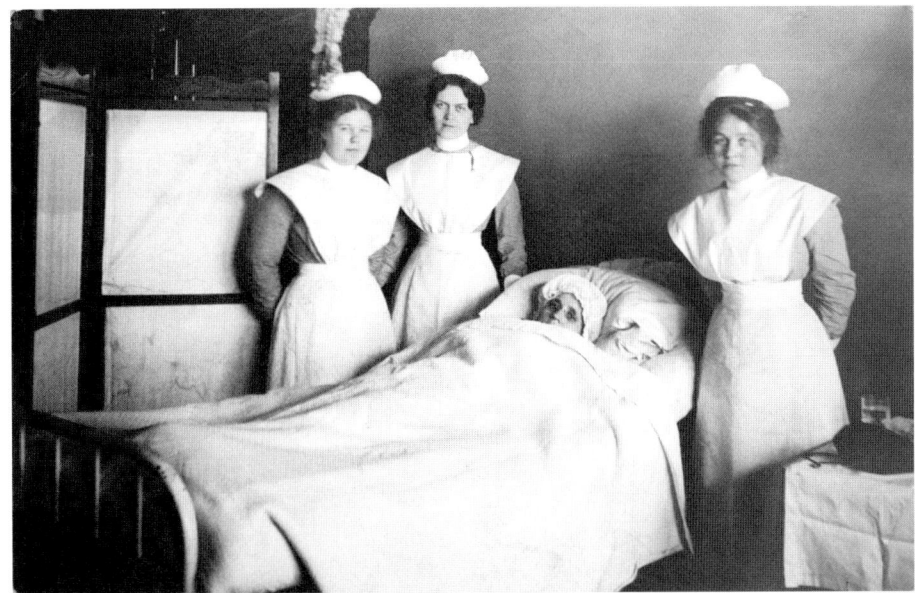

Right: Rachel Dahl, Mary Danielson, Katherine Stockfleth Hudson (all 1915)

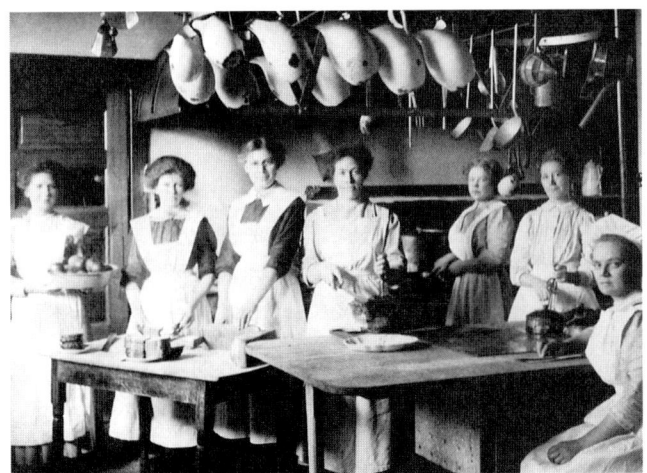

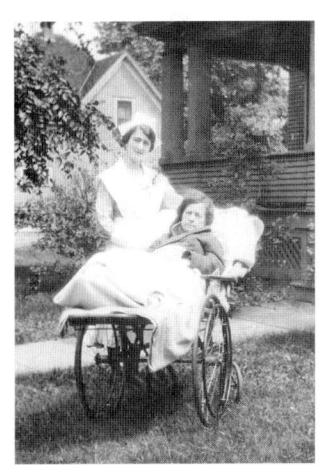

Above: With a patient, circa 1924

Above: Training in the Diet Kitchen, circa 1915.

Right: Patient's room, Mounds Park Sanitarium, 1908

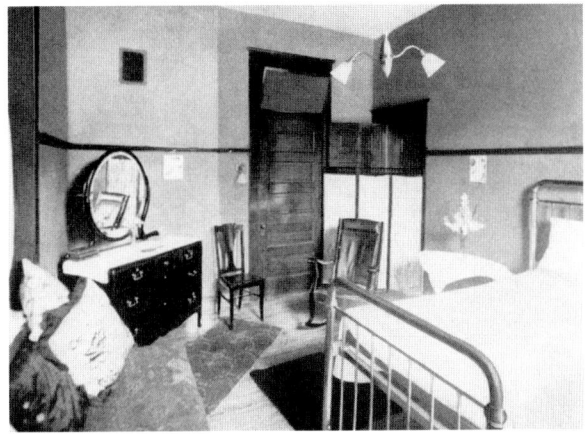

Chapter One 29

were aroused to a new sense of their dependence on the products of nursing schools, and many of them learned for the first time of the hopelessly limited resources which nursing educators have had to work with in the training of these indispensable servants.[20]

Growing Years

Mounds Park Sanitarium had proved to be an unqualified success. In 1917, a substantial addition opened, bringing capacity to 120 beds. Its professional reputation continued to grow, especially after Dr. Robert Earl spent a year in Europe, studying the latest advances in neurosurgery. He was now joined at Mounds by his younger brother, George.

However prolific new hospitals were in the Twin Cities, with their attendant nursing schools, there was no guarantee of success. On the opposite side of St. Paul, Cobb Hospital opened its doors at 2056 Iglehart in 1909. As was typical, they began a training school for nurses that same year. Primarily an obstetrical hospital, it had twenty-five beds, employed only one graduate nurse in 1913, and relied almost completely on its students. Because of this, the state board refused to accredit the program. In an attempt to bolster its standing, Cobb Hospital approved a one-year affiliation with the Hahnemann Hospital in Chicago. However, the state nursing board proved reluctant to give its approval. In 1920, with seven students, the school made plans to close.

In 1921, however, the Mounds Park board took over the institution's management, changing its name to the Merriam Park Hospital. They named Amelia Moen, a 1915 graduate, as superintendent, succeeded by Beth McCrank (1919) in 1923.

Nearby, the Midway General Hospital incorporated in 1912 with eighteen beds. It had a training school with only six students. Its management was apparently troubled because in 1916, the superintendent and twelve nurses left the hospital for some undisclosed reason. When the State Board of Examiners refused to recognize the training school, they sought affiliation with Mounds Park. However, Director Ruth Martin wrote back stating, "Our accommodations are somewhat limited as we are increasing our training this year."[21] Martin was right. With the additional hospital space, the school of nursing grew from forty-one students in 1917 to seventy-two in 1926.

Although rebuffed, within two years, however, the Mounds Park board decided to acquire the the Midway Hospital. With these new facilities, the old association officially changed its name to the Northwestern Baptist Hospital Association. The School of Nursing,

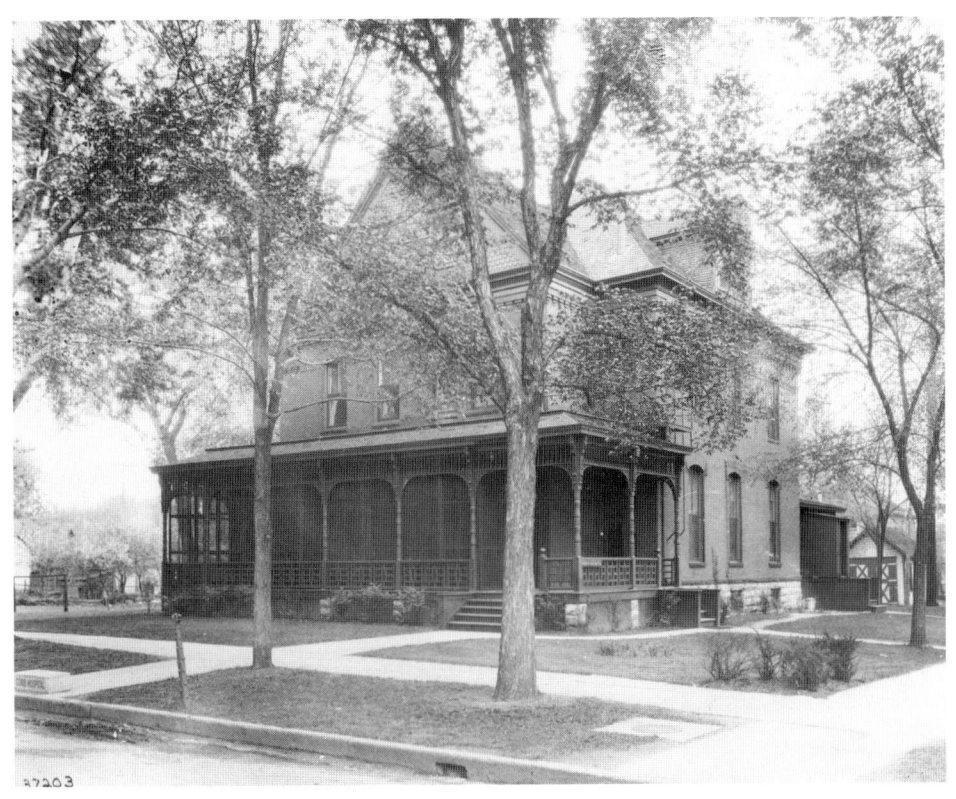

Above: The Association took over the Cobb Hospital on Iglehart Street in 1920 and operated it as the Merriam Park Hospital until it burned in 1925.

Right: The Mounds Park Hospital Association acquired the old Midway Hospital in 1920.

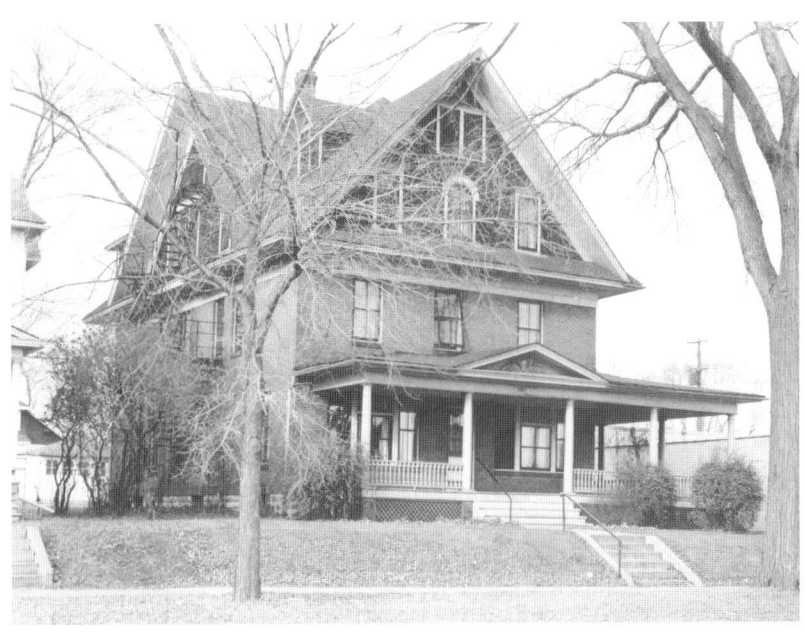

however, stuck to its identification, officially known as the Mounds School of Nursing.

The school was making great strides as an educational institution and a reviewer called Mounds, "One of the best conducted in the state." After 1917, when the National League of Nursing issued its landmark *Standard Curriculum for Schools of Nursing,* Mounds Park shifted its course work to reflect the new guidelines. The school increased the hours in the classroom from 232 hours in 1917 to 605 hours by 1926, conforming to the 595 hours recommended by the NLN. Work assignments used the following criteria:

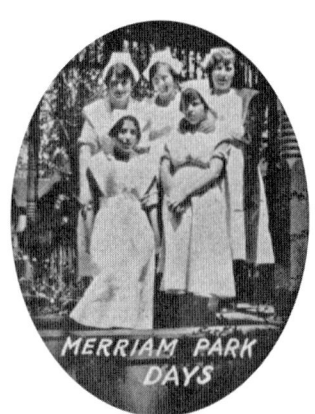

1. Night duty. Each nurse is allowed two terms of two months each.
2. Diet kitchen. Each nurse is allowed two terms of one and one-half months each in junior and intermediate years.
3. Special duty. Each nurse should have three months of special duty.
4. Obstetrical duty. Each nurse should have the care of at least five cases in the intermediate year.
5. Operating room, nine weeks; Dressing room, three weeks; Drug Room and Laboratory, three weeks.
6. Each nurse is given at least four months of head nursing if she seems qualified.

The postwar generation introduced a series of reforms in the educational system that raised the bar, beginning with the Goldmark report of 1923. Admission standards were raised, so that a high school diploma became essential by the end of the 1920s. National panels pressed for more laboratories and recommended the hiring of full-time teachers. A state nursing board reviewer, for example, noted one problem related to the school's expansion of campuses. Her report said:

The fact of the distance between the allied hospitals and the necessity for transferring the students back and forth for class work presents a difficulty which might be made easier with a full-time instructor who could go back and forth and save students time and strength.

This report strongly recommended that the school hire a full-time instructor, which it did in 1923. Maude Guest was a 1922 Mounds graduate, who taught high school prior to entry into the school. Following graduation, she took postgraduate classes at the University of Minnesota and worked as a night supervisor. After she left Saint Paul to teach at the Frances Willard Hospital in Chicago, she was replaced by Ruth Gustafson.

The New York Nursing Board, one of the most powerful in the country, also made several recommendations following an inspection visit in 1923. In obstetrics, its report stated, "There is not a graduate in charge of services." It also noted the lack of pediatric training and suggested that an affiliation be arranged with a nearby hospital.

This new generation of nursing students brought new attitudes with them. For example, the school administration expressed concern about the latest fashion, noting in 1920, "It was decided that an effort be made to prevent the nurses now in training from bobbing their hair and no probationers be admitted who have their hair bobbed."[22]

Student ledger, rotations, 1919

The catch phrases of the Jazz Age seeped into the vocabulary as well. To curb the bad habits, the residents of Hiawatha House, it was noted in 1923, "have installed a slang box, which demands one cent deposit for every slang word spoken. The sum is used in paying for the daily paper taken there, and the reminder of the amount is used for feeds."[23]

The newfound popularity of a career in nursing concerned a few administrators, especially when students left the school. A committee drafted a contract to be signed by students "in order to help students realize their duty in completing training and not resigning without adequate cause." Dr. Riggs, who was still on staff, warned,

> Nursing is not a trade. Nurses used to recognize this when they chose their calling. They knew they were not selecting a soft snap, an easy job, and they rejoiced in that knowledge. Only those who were willing to give more than was demanded became nurses. Nursing no less than medicine demands self-sacrifice as well as character and poise. I do not like to think that any large majority of the younger nurses are only thinking of how much they can make and how easy a time they can have.[24]

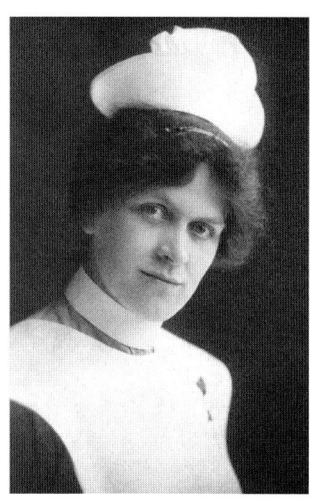

Mary Danielson as a student nurse at Mounds Park School of Nursing

Although there was considerable turnover in both staff and faculty, at the top, three key figures remained in charge. As Hazel Ahlstrom Addington (1918) noted, "With the passage of time many changes have been wrought both in personnel of the staff and faculty and in the institution itself. Dr. Robert, though he has grown a little farther up through his hair, is still the same. Dr. Riggs is his stately self. Dr. George evidently stood still long enough to have his picture taken but I am sure he was in a hurry."

The nursing school, in its first fifteen years, had seven directors: Caroline Monk, Ida Isaacson, Nora Tolbert (1909-1910), Ruth Martin (1910-1915, 1918-1919), Margaret Fortune, Alma Ryden (1918-1919), and Edith Thornquist (1919-1923). The revolving door halted, though, with the hiring of two Mounds graduates. Indeed, Mary Danielson and Ann Friedsburg would shape the hospital and school for the next three decades.

After growing up in Ely, Ann Friedsburg graduated from Mounds in 1918 and immediately became operating room supervisor.[25] With the acquisition of a new facility, Ann Friedsburg was offered the position as superintendent of the Midway Hospital in 1920. Despite her objections of inexperience, she took the post at the insistence of the Earls.

She recalled those early days at Midway, saying, "It was a three-and-a-half story building and had no elevator, no dumb waiter. Patients had to be carried up and down stairs. So did the meals. There were twelve student nurses, two graduate nurses, and later a night supervisor. We were on call at all times."[26]

Then, in 1923, Mary Danielson was named as director of the school of nursing. She graduated in the class of 1915, intending to follow in the footsteps of her namesake and aunt and become a missionary. Instead, she accepted an offer from Mounds to come work as night supervisor. She took increasing responsibility, working as the record librarian and sitting on the curriculum committee. Then came the appointment as Mounds Park Hospital administrator and director of the school of nursing. As a later biographical note said, "It seemed that God had other plans for her. He kept her at home. Crushed hopes did not make her bitter, however, nor did she turn from her interest in missions. Instead, as step by step, she followed God's leading, she entered into a wider usefulness for the very cause that was so dear to her."

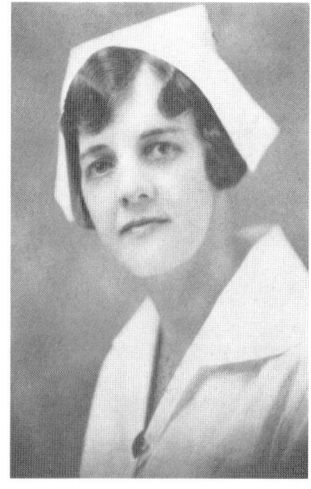

Ann Friedsburg in the 1920s

The Mounds School of Nursing, as it approached its third decade, was also entering a "wider usefulness." The profession had gained respectability and established itself as a career choice for young women. In Minnesota, for example, the number of people served by each trained nurse dropped dramatically from 956 in 1910 to 505 in 1920, falling to 298 in 1930. Nursing education had begun to formulate theories of training and took tentative steps toward the development of a curriculum.

In 1926, a fire severely damaged the Merriam Park Hospital. Discovered just as a Mrs. F. G. Hoelscher was wheeled into the operating room "where the stork was to meet her," the superintendent, Esther Erickson, hailed a passing motorist and had the prospective mother rushed to Midway. "Stork Nearly Singed in Hospital Flames," read the headline in the *St. Paul Dispatch*. The hospital board decided not to re-open Merriam Park and soon sold the lot.

By this time, a new hospital was on the drawing boards.

Endnotes

[1] David A. Lanegran, "Swedish Neighborhoods of the Twin Cities," in *Swedes in the Twin Cities: Immigrant Life and Minnesota's Urban Frontier*, Philip J. Anderson and Dag Blanck, ed. (St. Paul: Minnesota Historical Society Press, 2001), 40-49.

[2] *Brief Record of the History of the Payne Avenue Baptist Church* (Saint Paul: 1948), 19.

[3] "Robert O. Earl," *Minnesota Medicine*, 32 (March 1949), 296.

[4] Dr. George Earl, "A Brother's Tribute," *Mounds-Midway News Letter*, 13 (December 1948), 2. Also see Steven E. Koop, *We Hold This Treasure: The Story of the Gillette Children's Hospital* (Afton, Minn.: Afton Historical Society Press, 1998), 25-30.

[5] *Baptist Hospital Bulletin,* I (May-June 1957), 3.

[6] *The Mounds Park Sanitarium Association*, 1906.

[7] *A Memorial Sketch of the First Swedish Baptist Church, Saint Paul, Minnesota* (1923), 38-39.

[8] *The Mounds Park Sanitarium Association*, 1906.

[9] C. Eugene Riggs, "Reminiscences," *Minnesota Medicine,* January 1928, 1-11.

[10] Monk resigned after one year, possibly to be married. See U.S. Census, 1900, and St. Paul City Directory, 1902.

[11] Application, Jennie Teberg, MMSN Alumni Association Museum.

[12] Jennie Teberg Paquette, "An Eyewitness Account," Mounds Midway News Letter (1957). 3-4.

[13] School Record Book. Minnesota Historical Society.

[14] *The Gong* (St. Paul: Mounds-Midway School of Nursing, 1928), 85. Martin later became Superintendent of the City Hospital in Red Wing, Minnesota.

[15] *Mounds-Midway Nurses Alumnae Association Bulletin* (May 1941), 33; Adella Espelien, *A History of the Mounds-Midway School of Nursing* (St. Paul, Minn.:1967), 13.

[16] Instruction Sheet for Pupil Nurses, Mounds Park Sanitarium of Nursing, 1915. Mounds-Midway Alumni Association Museum.

[17] *The Gong* (1928), 28.

[18] Minnesota State Board of Examiners of Nursing Report, 1910. Minnesota Historical Society.

[19] *Baptist Hospital Bulletin,* I (May-June 1957), 3.

[20] Isabel M. Stewart, *Developments in Nursing Education Since 1918* (1921).

[21] Correspondence, Mounds School of Nursing, 14 April 1917, 25 May 1918. State Nursing Board, Minnesota Historical Society.

[22] Quoted in Adella Espelien, *A History of Mounds-Midway School of Nursing* (St. Paul: Mounds-Midway Alumni Association, 1967), 9.

[23] *The Mound Builder,* I (1 February 1923).

[24] C. Eugene Riggs, *Minnesota Medicine* (January 1928), 1-11.

[25] *The Gong* (1928), 92.

[26] Falsum Russell, "Midway Hospital Builder to Quit after 42 Years," *St. Paul Pioneer Press*, 1962.

CHAPTER TWO

To Be a Nurse

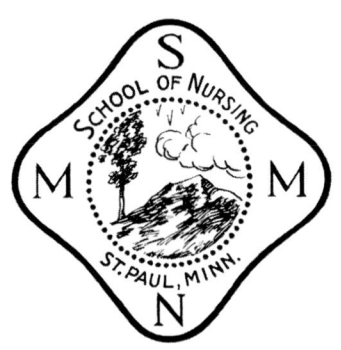

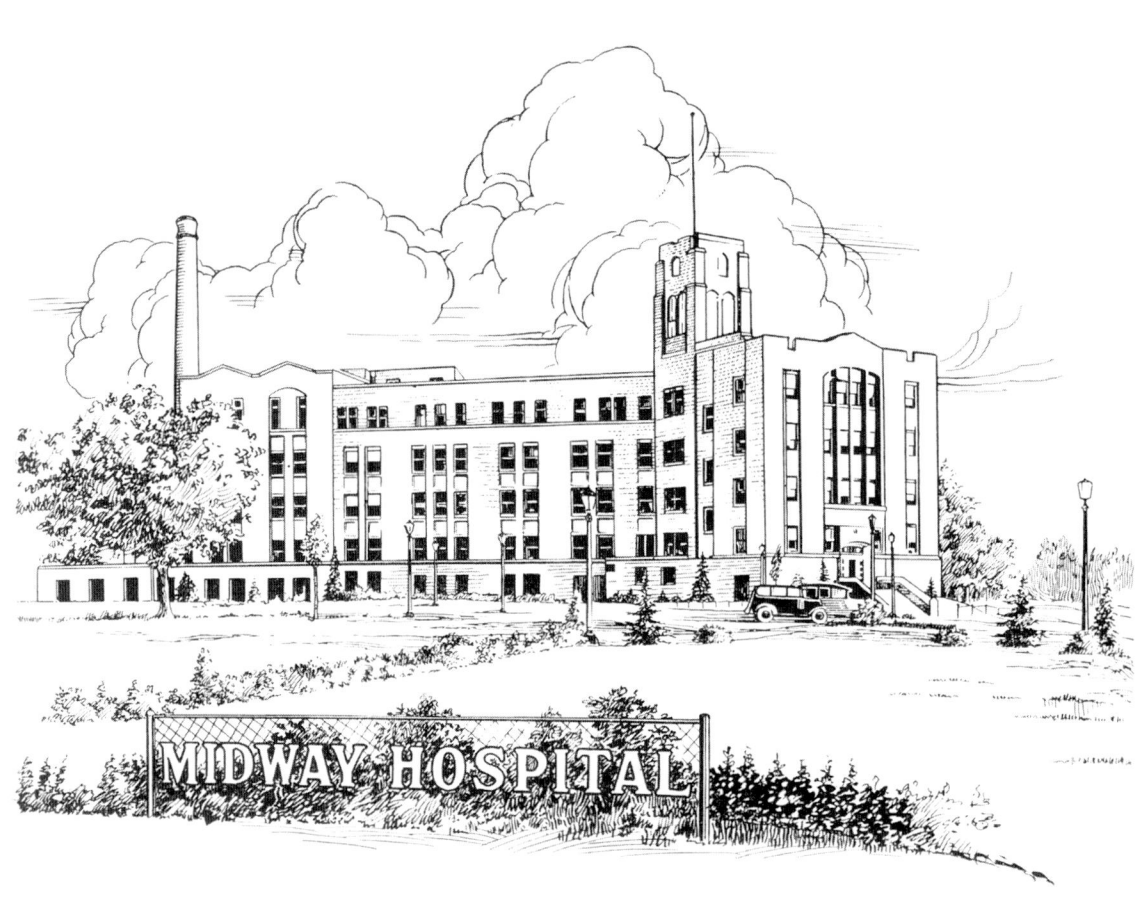

*T*HE MIDWAY AREA, AS the name suggests, sits halfway between downtown Saint Paul and Minneapolis—still with open fields in the 1920s, but filling rapidly with small homes and shops along University, Snelling, Marshall, and Selby Avenues. The Midway Club, a local business booster organization, heavily promoted the district for new industrial and commercial investment. "It has unusual transportation facilities, room for trackage, and or plant expansion," stated one promotional article. "Radiating lines from the Midway touch the rim of the earth."

Mounds Park Hospital had been eyeing expansion into the neighborhood for several years, first with the acquisition of Midway Hospital in December 1919. At the same time, the Association purchased a wooded eight-acre site fronting on University Avenue. One year later, the newly-organized Midway Hospital Company—Drs. Robert and George Earl, directors—purchased the twenty-bed Cobb Hospital. Led by Dr. George Earl, the Northwestern Baptist Hospital Association—the new name for the combined hospitals—initiated a Capital Fund drive among denominational members in seven states. The appeal to churches read: "These are the only [hospitals] owned by the Baptists of the Northwest. This work adds to the church activities, the most practical expression of the Christian religion,—that the love alleviating suffering, which is a constant contribution to the advancement of the kingdom."[1]

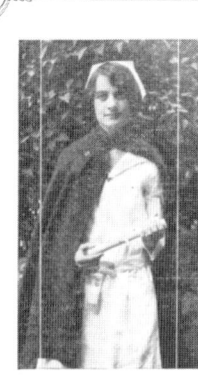

The Northwestern Baptist Hospital Association highlighted the role of its nurse graduates when appealing for donations. The woman is Edna Pearson Holm (1929).

The businessmen of the Midway community agreed to assist and raised one dollar for every two dollars donated by the Baptists. The hospital was a good investment, claimed one letter to Midway Club members, since it would be "almost at the geographic center of this industrial area with its population of 78,000 people and over 200 industrial plants. . . . Not an industry, but a most certain and definite actor in keeping the manpower of the industrial world efficient."[2]

On July 1, 1925, a contract was awarded for the erection of a modern hospital with 135 beds, costing three-quarters of a million dollars. "I saw it go up from the start," Ann Friedsburg remembered. Dr. George Earl wanted her to be so familiar with the building that he even insisted that she know the entire plumbing layout, location of the steam pipes,

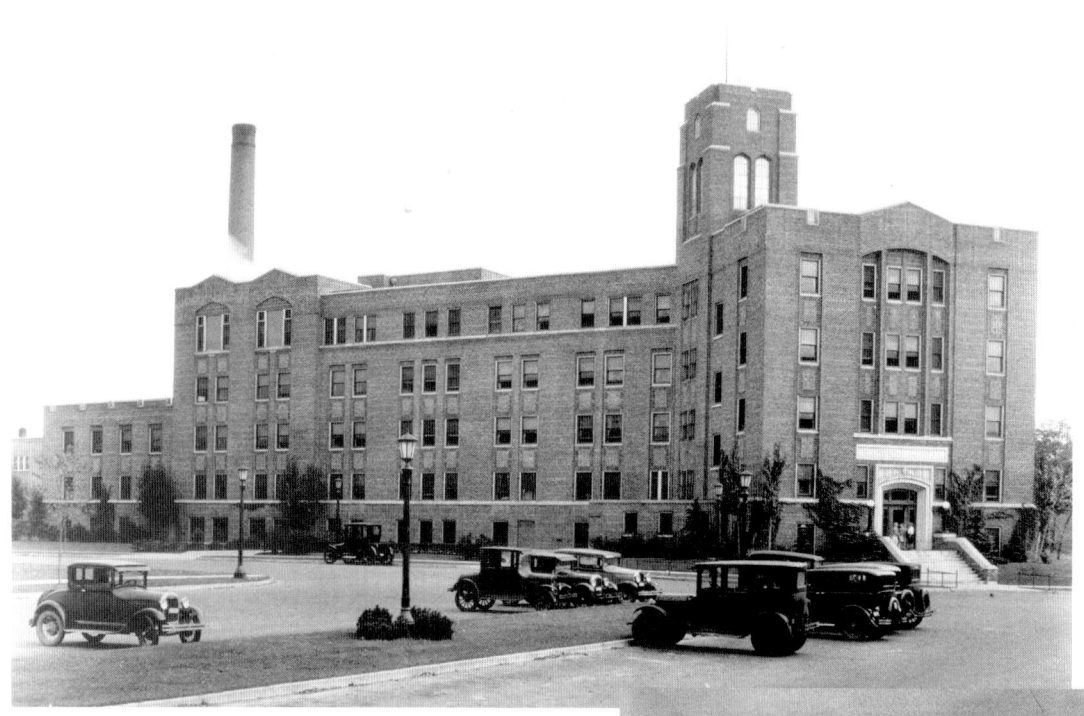

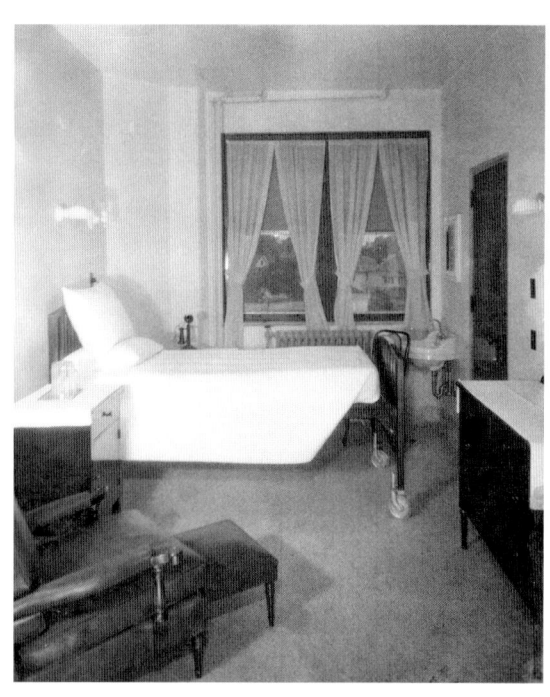

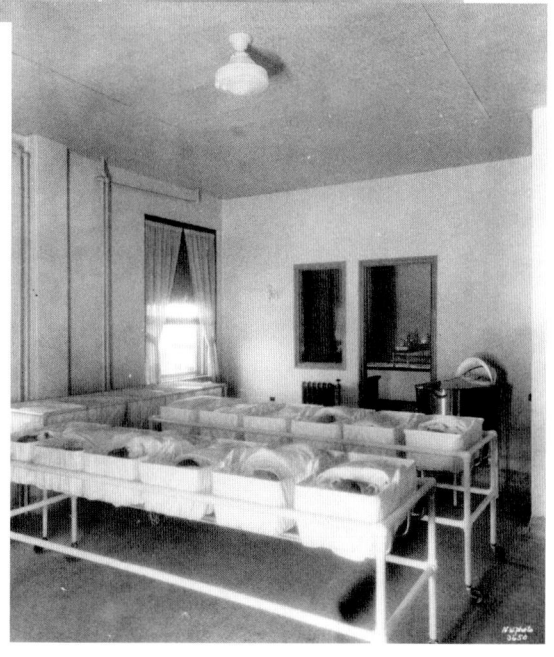

Midway Hospital, 1926. Left: Patient's room. Above: Nursery.

and all. She also was in charge of getting the specifications out and soliciting bids.³

The new Midway Hospital was magnificent with state-of-the-art facilities. A brochure, describing the hospital, noted the following features

> a lovely reception room for guests furnished in brown and Spanish leather, private rooms with separate bath in double doors to keep out all sound, adjustable beds and steel furniture; light signal systems; telephone and radio service in private rooms; lights above the bed, walls and floors of the operating room with orchid light-absorbing tile; microscopic and chemical laboratories adjacent to the operating suite; soundproof delivery rooms and nursery; x-ray rooms with fluoroscopic and deep therapy equipment; service rooms with automatic dumb waiters; and the reception room in the nurses quarters has been given every comfort.

With the hospital opening in 1926, the school officially changed its name to the Mounds-Midway School of Nursing, and welcomed thirty-one new pupils, all high school graduates, on August 10, 1926. Some students moved into a new dorm on Aldine Street, known as the "Cottage," although all teaching was done at Mounds for the first few years.

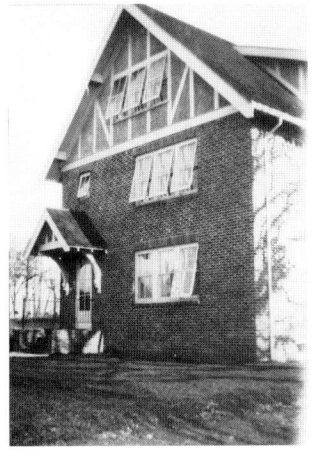

The Cottage on Aldine Street

Leadership

The principal leadership of the Hospital Association and the School of Nursing was in place and remained there for the next two decades. Dr. Robert Earl continued to be the guiding spirit, but now shared much of the responsibility with his younger brother, George.

Although Ann Friedsburg had less to do with teaching the student nurses, her presence was everywhere. Mel Conley, longtime administrator, remembered his early impressions of her when he came to Mounds-Midway in 1946:

> Back in 1946 she not only lived in the hospital, but she worked from seven a.m. to seven p.m., six days a week. She hired all of the professional staff and kept records of their time for payroll purposes. She scheduled all of the surgery. She admitted all patients and assigned their rooms. She purchased the medical supplies and equipment. She supervised the business office and she still had

Chapter Two 41

time to make rounds on a daily basis to be sure that the patients were having all of their needs met and to give encouragement to members of the staff.

The Northwestern Baptist Hospital Association added another important staff member when it hired a young accountant named Arthur Calvin to serve as manager.

Of course, Mary Danielson was the heart and soul of the nursing school. Her personality provided calm, steady direction. Florence Jacobson Berlin, who graduated in 1929, remembered a class taken under Mary Danielson, writing, "I will always remember our class in ethics, the things you taught us, to be a good credit to our nursing profession, and to keep up the standards of our school."

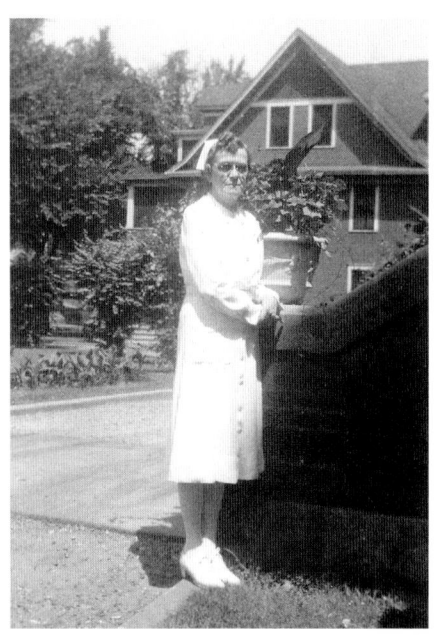

Mary Danielson

Always fair. That phrase echoes through memories shared with Miss Danielson on her twenty-fifth anniversary in the job. "A characteristic that appeals to me," Violet Nelson wrote, "is your ability to be so fair, and to give the other fellow the benefit of the doubt. When some of the rest of us would have been impatient, just this one quality in itself helped create the sense of loyalty manifested in the people working at Mounds in the great respect and admiration that the students have always shown for you."

Irene Smith seconded this opinion, saying, "Even the visits we made to your office on your request weren't so bad. You're always fair, and as I remember I was pretty good at presenting my own side of the issue. I have to smile though when I think of the way my knees shook."

There was a respect for her ability to gently correct the students. Bernice Thorson Lemon (1947) remembered, "My gross error as a student nurse [was] giving a double dose of morphine by syringe. My honest confession, bright and early, to Superintendent Danielson, lightened my discipline to an in-depth report on "The Dosage and Use of Morphine" in front of *all* my classmates.

Gwendolyn Ticknor (1934) recalled another difficult encounter:

> Once, I remember how hurt I was when you failed to notify me that I was off night duty. Friends came and begged me to take a trip. And I said I should be off night duty, but guess I am not, because I have not been notified. My friends left. I dressed for duty, and

went to the floor to get the report and found out I'd been off nights the entire day. Too angry to cry, I went to your office and blew off. You were so surprised that you never said a word until I finished, and then, without raising your voice said, "Miss Ticknor, I am just as sorry." Feeling you were very sincere, I dismissed the matter and had a grand weekend, in love with you more than ever.

Under the leadership of Mary Danielson, the school saw generation follow generation in the nursing profession. Effie Ostergrew, who graduated in the class of 1914, reminisced with Mary Danielson. "I remember the time I was in charge of third floor," she said, "and you were one of my nurses. I never had to worry when I assigned some work to you, that it would be well done." In turn, Effie's daughter, Ruth, became a nurse as well.

There was a key addition in 1925, when Ruth Gustafson joined the faculty. She was a graduate of the Swedish Hospital School of Nursing in Minneapolis, and had recently completed postgraduate work in nursing education at Columbia University in New York.

If Mary Danielson was fair, Ruth Gustafson was remembered as kind by students and fellow workers. Danielson wrote about her: "She began as an instructor in the days when one instructor was responsible for the teaching of many subjects, and there are many alumni who remember her patience as they learned the names of the bones of the body in Anatomy, or as they strove to master the art of Materia Medica. As the faculty increased the number, more and more of the administration work was delegated to her, and she emerged finally as the Educational Director with the task of coordinating the educational activities of the entire school and its faculty."[4]

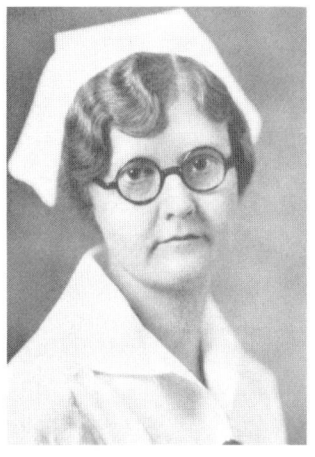

Ruth Gustafson

Depression

As America tumbled into the depths of the Depression, it began to have a disastrous effect on Mounds and Midway Hospitals. Throughout the 1920s, hospitals expanded bed capacity, but as the economy collapsed, sick people avoided medical care.

Mounds-Midway had just completed a major capital campaign to finance the building of its new hospital. By early 1933, patients' hospital accounts fell drastically behind and pledges by wealthy donors were not being paid. Average patient occupancy dropped from 200 per day in 1930 to 143 per day in 1933. The Northwest Baptist Hospital Association tried to work out an agreement with its bondholders. Yet in the end, several brought suit and the Board of Directors reluctantly placed the association into a receivership. Salaries were cut and staff was laid off, in order to bring the budget into balance.[5]

In the nursing school, student allowances were cut to two dollars in 1929, and then dropped completely in 1930. Although there was no tuition, the school began charging an entrance fee of $15 and a general fee in 1934 of $66 to cover the cost of uniforms, medical examinations, and laboratory fees. The first official tuition fee was not charged until 1941.[6]

There was also a sharp drop in the school's enrollment, falling from a high of 114 in 1928 down to a low of only sixty-one in 1934. That year, only one class was admitted, partly in response to the recommendation of national nursing organizations to relieve the unemployment situation among graduate nurses. Mary Danielson wrote, "Since this measure was carried out by the average school throughout the country, many small schools were closed. A definite shortage of nurses has resulted in many localities." In fact, the number of accredited schools in Minnesota dropped from fifty in 1931 to thirty-seven in 1934.

Arthur Calvin looked for a creative approach to stabilize hospital income. After the stock market crash of 1929, physicians and hospitals sought a steady flow of income upon which they could base their planning and operating decisions. Patients wanted the security of knowing that they could receive care when they needed it and that it would not devastate them financially. In 1931, Calvin attended the annual meeting of the American Hospital Association, at which an experimental group health plan was presented, tried on a small scale at Baylor Hospital in Texas. In return for an annual payment of six dollars per year, the enrolled members received a guarantee of coverage for hospital care. It covered up to twenty-one days of care at Baylor and included operating room service, anesthetics, and laboratory fees.

Taking the idea back to the Twin Cities, Calvin and Dr. Peter Ward, of Miller Hospital, brought together seven St. Paul Hospital administrators and designed a prepayment plan, announcing it in December 1932 in *Minnesota Medicine*. The concept was immediately popular. As a marketing tool to identify the Hospital Service Association's literature in 1934, they adopted a blue cross, a symbol of relief for those struck by disaster. Calvin was the board's secretary until 1939 when he was appointed to the position of executive director, ending his days at Mounds Midway. By the time of his death in his beloved Midway Hospital in 1957, Blue Cross subscribers numbered one-and-a-half million.[7]

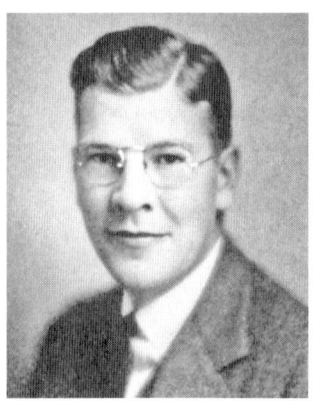

Arthur Calvin was the executive director of the Northwestern Baptist Hospital Association and a founder of Blue Cross.

The Education of a Nurse

There was still an inherent tension in the basic structure of a nursing school. On one hand, the hospital wished to maintain an inexpensive, somewhat malleable, work force. Counter that, on the national level, professional nursing organizations played an increasingly vocal role in raising the training school standards and demanding a clearer division between the hospital's needs and the student's best interests. Isabel Stewart lamented: "It has cost the public practically nothing to produce the hundreds of thousands of nurses who have spent their lives in its service. Nurses have paid for their own education, and through their services have contributed . . . millions of dollars toward the care of the sick in hospitals."[8] An influential 1934 report, *Nursing Schools — Today and Tomorrow* — stated, "Hospitals are not schools; and despite the many advantages it offers, working as an apprentice in a hospital is not the same as studying in a school."[9]

And yet, for the hundreds of young students who entered the school, it seemed a golden opportunity. Many came from rural families, where post-secondary education was rare, especially among women. It offered an education at little expense.

Mounds-Midway tried to keep pace with the national standards, as Mary Danielson noted in 1936: "Indication that nursing education has steadily progressed in our school is evidenced by the fact that approximately 375 hours of class work has been added to the nursing course in the past ten years, the total number of hours now being 975. The National League of Nursing Education recommends a total of 1200 hours." To allow more time for studying, work hours dropped from nine to eight hours per day.[10]

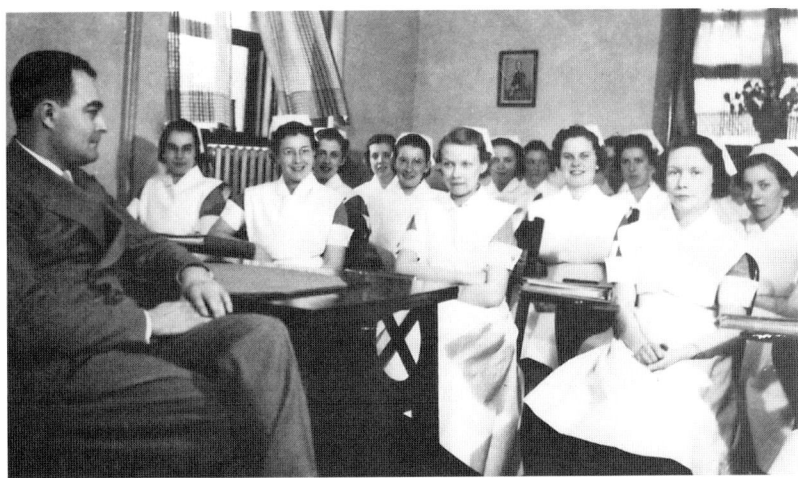

Obstetrics lecture, late 1930s.

1938 Curriculum

PRELIMINARY AND FIRST YEAR

Nursing Practice	130	Chemistry	32
History of Nursing	30	Ethics	20
Personal Hygiene	15	Foods and Nutrition	45
Bacteriology	30	Massage	12
Elem. Anatomy & Physiology	30	Psychology	30
Elem. Materia Medica	20	Bible Study	15
Emergency and First Aid	15		

FIRST YEAR

Advanced Nursing Practice	30	Surg. Technique	12
Pathology	20	Case Study Methods	10
Adv. Anatomy & Physiology	70	Obstetrics	30
Diet in Disease	15		

JUNIOR

Surgery and Gynecology	30	Public Hygiene & Sanitation	10
Surgical Nursing	15	Materia Medica	30
Medical Diseases	20	Neuropsychiatric Nursing	15
Dermatology	10	Communicable Diseases	10
Tuberculosis	10	Eye, Ear, Nose, Throat, Teeth	15
Child Guidance	5	Occupational Therapy	10

SENIOR

Public Health	12	Neuropsychiatry	15
Professional Problems	30	Pediatrics: includes Principles of Ped. Nursing Diseases of Children Communicable Diseases Orthopedic Conditions Child Psychology Infant Feedings Clinical Ward Teaching	110

In 1933, the school hired Caroline Krueger — a graduate of Mounds-Midway (1929) and Wheaton College — and its first faculty member with a baccalaureate degree. A few years later, she married and moved to California. For her replacement, the faculty gained a new teacher who would prove to be an institutio — Violet Nelson. She had graduated from the University of California with a degree in secondary education. After teaching high school for several years, she came to Mounds-Midway as a student, and upon graduation in 1936, became a member of the faculty.

Other significant changes to the faculty included the addition of Amy Johnson as the first full-time instructor at Midway Hospital in 1936. She lasted only one year, but was replaced by Annette Grandin, a 1934 graduate of Swedish Covenant Hospital in Chicago. If Mary Danielson was distant at times, Annette Grandin could be warm and encouraging. She was, said, June Evers Benson (1947), "the nurse I wanted to be just like. She always . . . conducted herself as a true professional nurse."

The Mounds-Midway experience began with tentative steps, as the young women, some in the big city for the first time in their lives, entered the hospital. It meant donning the black stockings and shoes of the probie, as Janice Faelske Binning recalled, "People thought I was entering a convent to be a nun."

Bernice Franck Swanson (1933) wrote, "A long time has passed since that February day. I found myself nervously waiting in the reception at Mounds Park Hospital. Now as I look back, I know that, that day can be counted as one of the most important days of my life. To try to explain in words, what Mounds-Midway has meant, and still means, would be futile, but as I've worked in many places, I've said many a time, 'Thank God, I was sent to Mounds Midway.'"

Alice Olson (1931) wrote: "My spring classmates and I entered nursing training at Mounds Park Hospital on February 7, 1928. We were a mixed group of high school graduates. A few had been in the work force in the city. The others came from small towns or daughters of farm parents. It was a new life for a close knit group of teenagers. Under Mary Danielson's guidance, we were well watched physically, spiritually, and urged to work hard. We were the mop personnel, furniture movers, etc. It was a ten-hour day which often ended up to be eleven or twelve hours."[11]

First-year students were placed in the hands of two women for their early training. Looking at the 1938 curriculum, of the 988 hours,

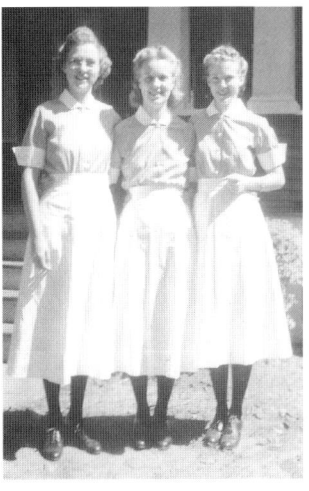

Probies, 1946

We wore black stockings and black shoes during our six month probationary period. Oh, how we hated getting dressed in the morning in those garter belts and black stockings!
Ardis Williamson Denner (1946)

160 — roughly fifteen percent of all instruction — was given by Violet Nelson in two Nursing Arts classes. Ruth Gustafson taught a similar number of hours but covering subjects as psychology, the history of nursing, and anatomy and physiology. Many of the classes were led by staff physicians, including both Dr. Earls, Dr. Kvitrud in pathology, and Drs. James Swendson and Walter in obstetrics. Of course, much of the instruction took place in the wards under the tutelage of staff nurses.

Nursing Arts was the introduction to the profession, with the stated purpose to: "prepare the students to meet problems that will confront them in their daily work in the hospital and to test the attitude of the students as to their fitness to continue their training as nurses." Upon entering the school, beginning in 1936, the first-year students were handed into the care of Miss Violet Nelson — a petite woman who spoke with absolute authority. She heartily accepted the challenge to test the attitudes of young women and shape them into her vision of what a nurse should be. Ardis Williamson Denner (1946) remembered, "Miss Nelson insisted that we should act and speak like ladies. We were told to address each other as Miss Larson, Miss Johnson, Miss Mettner, Miss Mundheim, Miss Samuelson." Of course, her class chose to go by nicknames instead, "Even after all these years we are known as Jamie, Larsie, Sigie, Metty, Mundy, Sammy, and Willie."

Apart from the class work, probies were expected to master mundane tasks and work long hours. Lucille Walter Reed (1943) recalled, "Our probie days [began] at six, chapel at six-thirty, and on the way to chapel

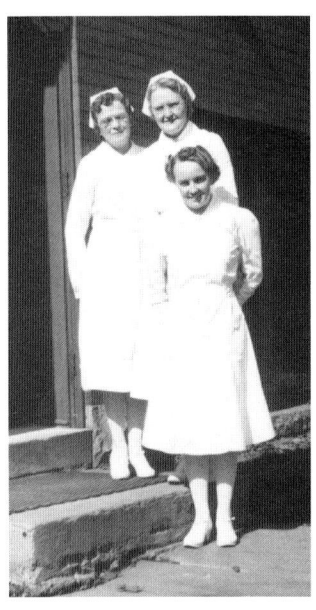

Three women set the tone for the School of Nursing during the era: Mary Danielson, Ruth Gustafson, and Violet Nelson

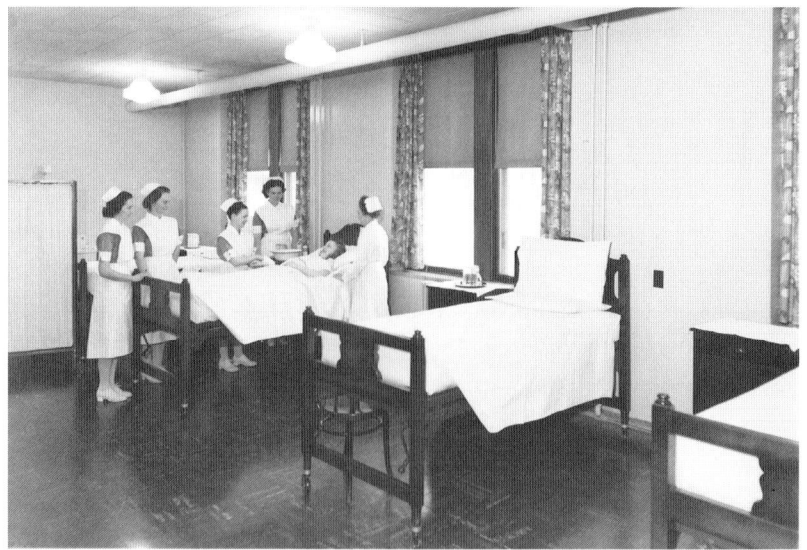

The Nursing Arts lab

we encountered our house mother at the foot of the stairs, checking us over. Black shoes polished, uniforms clean and neat, no jewelry, no long nails, not too much make up. On the nursing stations, we began by scrubbing linen closets, bathrooms, utility rooms, and they were given the white glove test. Before the four months of probie days ended, we proficiently were doing patient care: baths and back rubs were our expertise."[12]

Because Mounds had no sinks or toilets in the patient rooms, much of the early training meant carrying water back and forth. It also required the emptying of bedpans, neatly covered with a cloth as one walked down the hall. "It was such an embarrassment to meet someone while carrying a pan," wrote Helen Sammons Grooms (1942). A friend's advice cured her: "Phyllis Gagstetter just told me to pretend it was FDR's."

Bernice Thorson Lemon (1947) remembered that early introduction to nursing, saying, "There were many firsts: cleaning bathrooms to enemas, making a bed with a patient in it, and, at last, to give a live person a bed bath! Our first postoperative patient, who was so very nauseated, reminds me of a sympathetic Dagne Sondrol Christenson (1947). I found her one day under the patient's bed, joining him in his nauseous vomiting experience."

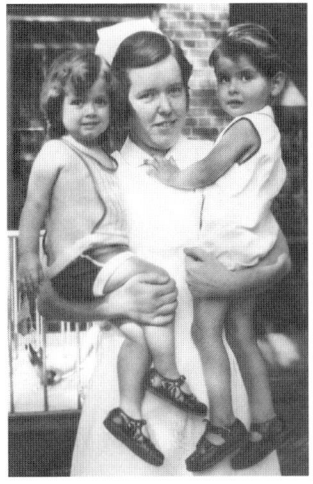

Dorothy Soderberg (1932) at Children's Hospital

One of the changes that took place in the 1930s, based on a recommendation of the State Board, was to add an affiliation with Children's Hospital. Pediatric training had been encouraged by the Red Cross and required for those wishing to enter their service. It began in 1929, and, except a one-year interruption in 1933 when the rotation shifted to Gillette Hospital, continued for several decades. It opened the door for new medical experiences for the students, but also new emotional ones as well. One student wrote, "We shall never forget some of our dear little patients, which were our privilege to care for during their stay. They will linger in our memories."

Gladys Thorson Newman (1940) recalled a few of those memories. She had been assigned the care of three children under the age of two, one with a severe case of diarrhea. The first step was to clean up this little boy. Next was to check the bandages of a child recovering from a mastoidectomy. She sat, giving formula to a third child whose parents had left her to go off on vacation, when the head nurse came in and said, "Miss Thorson, I just checked your last two patients. They are a mess. The diarrhea patient is covered in bowel movement and your

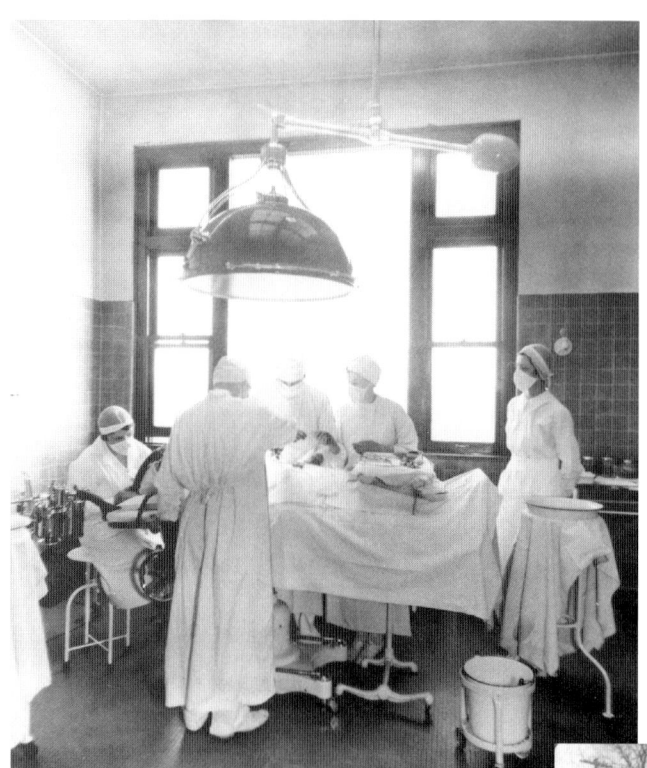
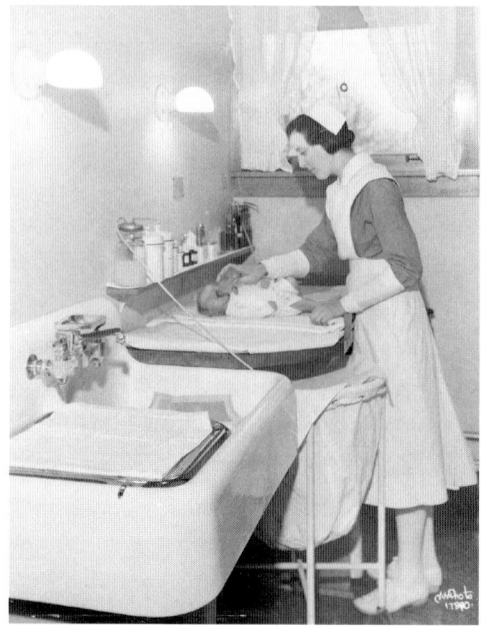
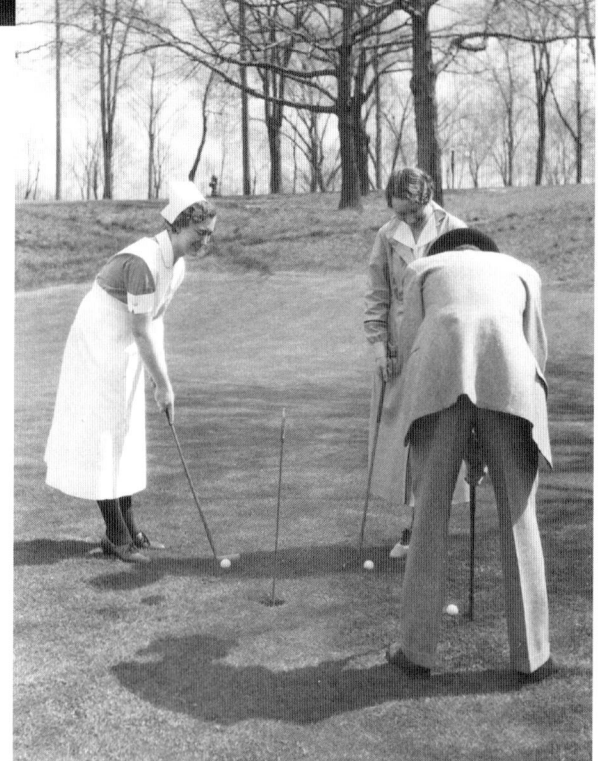

Nursing in the 1930s

Above, left: Dr. Earl in the new surgery room at Midway Hospital.

Above right: Student nurse in 1932. MHS

Right: Student nurses often took the psychiatric patients outdoors. Mounds Park Hospital maintained a putting green.

mastoid patient just tore all her bandages off." She was glad when the day was over.[13]

Work in the psychiatric unit at Mounds Park remained a vital part of the student's training. "Two floors were designated for the mental patients," recalled Helen Sammons Grooms (1942), "ranging from good rooms, which had nicer linens, dishes, silverware, and food trays, to the Annex where all patients were strapped to their beds in full restraint." Student tasks included taking patients on walks, giving sedative baths, and wrapping them in hot packs.

Summarizing the academic changes during these years, Ruth Gustafson wrote, "The trend has been that of elevating the standards for the school and to give the student the best possible preparation. . . . A more careful selection of students has been emphasized and many applicants have had some college preparation before entrance." The State Board of Examiners surveyed the school in 1939, and in their report, made several pointed recommendations, imploring them to build a science laboratory for the teaching of microbiology and anatomy. In response, the ground floor at Mounds Park was converted into classrooms and offices. One of the classrooms was equipped as a science laboratory and the library was expanded. The reviewers also decried the inadequate bathrooms at Mounds Park Hospital, and expressed a wish for a reorganization of the training school committee to include at least one, preferably two, lay women.[14]

Encouraged by a steady series of improvements, the school applied for national accreditation from the National League of Nursing in 1940. Although unsuccessful, it shows that the staff and the board of directors, led by the Earls still tried to hold Mounds-Midway up to the highest professional standards.[15]

The Life of a Student Nurse

"In many ways, our dorm was like a cloister," wrote Helen Sammons Grooms. "We shared experiences with life and death, together."

In the first months, the student was on probation and making the grade consumed most of their waking hours. Four months later, the

"AN EARNED REST AND REHABILITATION"
Missionaries, ministers and workers on the foreign field of service have break-downs often from their strenuous tasks. They need medical care, comfort and rehabilitation so that they may obtain their desire to go back and finish the task.

There was still a stigma associated with mental health illnesses. This image tried to overcome that by showing that even ministers and missionaries might need medical care and rehabilitation.

Chapter Two 51

Student Life, 1930s

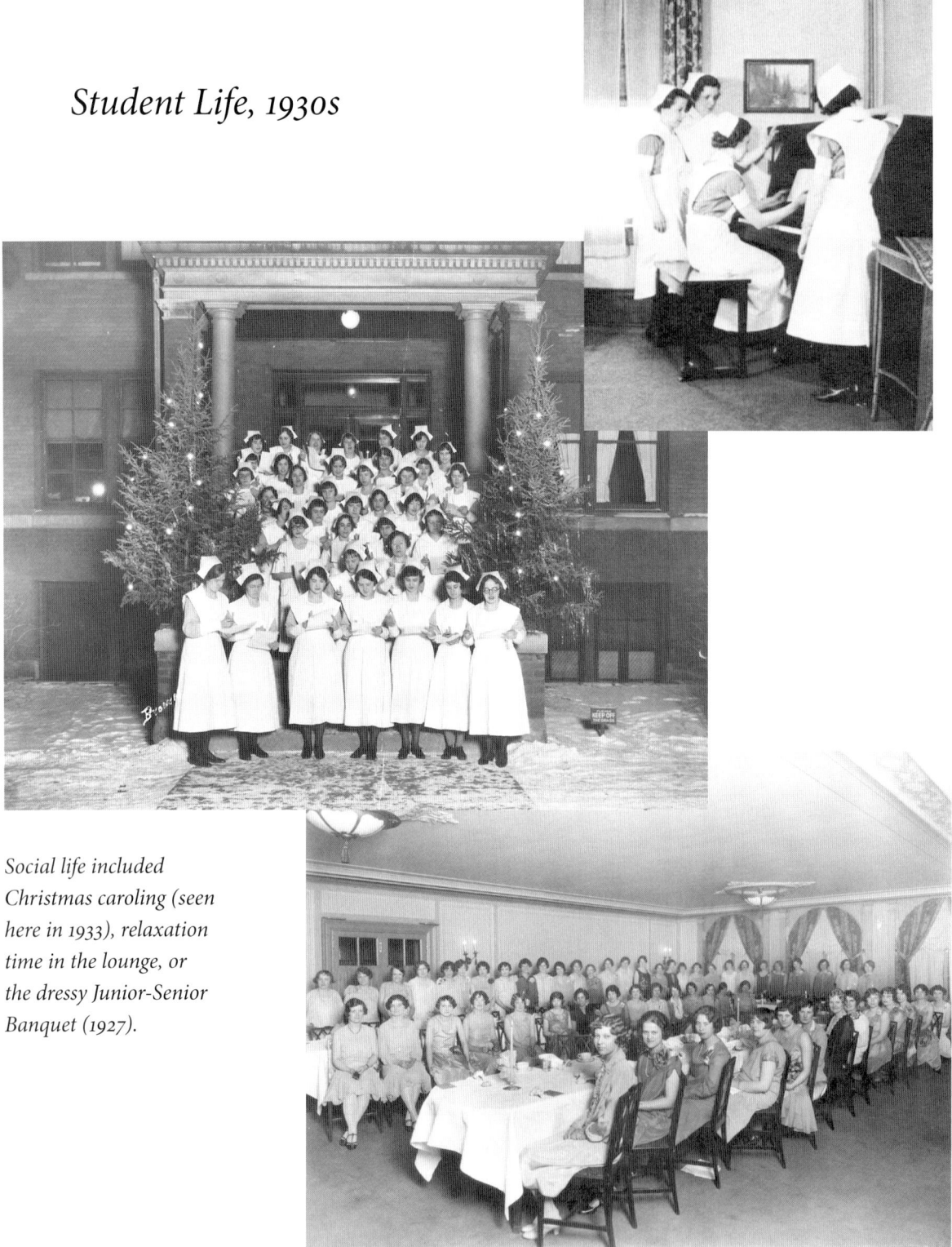

Social life included Christmas caroling (seen here in 1933), relaxation time in the lounge, or the dressy Junior-Senior Banquet (1927).

52 THIS CAP OF WHITE

probationary period ended. As one student described those days in 1938: "May 30: Gee, to pack or not to pack—accepted or not accepted. June 3: Accepted—wire. telephone, or write the news. I wonder if the building ever heard so many knees knock? June 13: We arrived at the first milestone. Received our caps and bibs with some difficulty in retaining our equilibrium."

On January 24, 1928, twenty-nine preliminary students gathered for the first evening capping ceremony. Opening remarks by Mary Danielson and Ruth Gustafson emphasized that in order to be successful in their chosen profession, the young students needed to possess the spirit of great nursing leaders, especially Florence Nightingale. Then, seniors marched to the podium, followed by a roll call, and each first-year student came forward and received their prized white cap from Miss Danielson. This tradition, a moment when the student entered the sisterhood of white-capped nurses, continued to hold emotional resonance throughout the remaining years of the school.[16]

Although students remained busy, working long days and studying during off-hours, they also had a social life. Before the war, three social events broke up the doldrums of the school year—a Halloween party, a Christmas dinner, and a Valentine's Day banquet. At Christmas, the students, carrying lighted candles, went down the halls and sang Christmas carols.

A favorite way to relieve the tension of classes and work was to spend time outdoors. As one student wrote: "Our class donned our hiking clothes and walked to Battle Creek. By the blazing fire we roasted wieners and marshmallows. We have spent many an hour at Battle Creek since we came and love it very much."

And they were still young and full of life. One only has to read between the lines of this piece of whimsy, published in the 1932 *Gong*—a yearbook named after the dreaded six a.m. bell—to guess some typical student activities.

Our Ten Commandments
1. Thou shalt strip thy bed on set date, lest thou bathe in vain.
2. Thou shalt not call the kitchen for malted milks, lest Miss Heaberlin answers.
3. Thou shalt not hide from devotions, lest Miss Thorne finds thee.
4. Thou shalt treat the seniors with respect, that it may be well in the days of thy training.

Dorm Life, 1930s

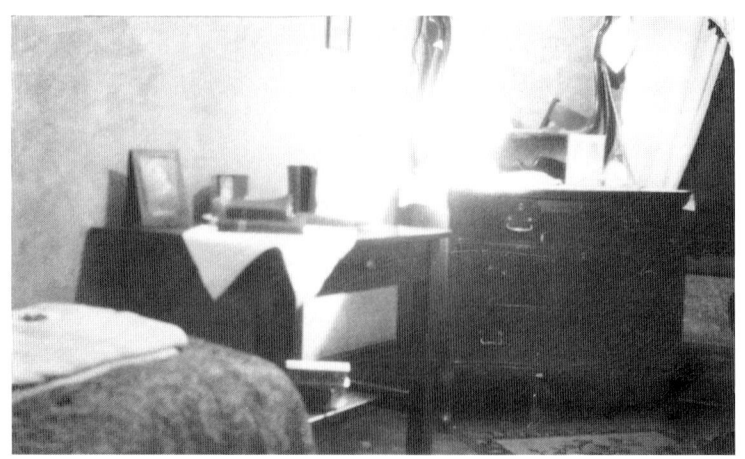

Dorm room in 222 Earl Street, circa 1926-27

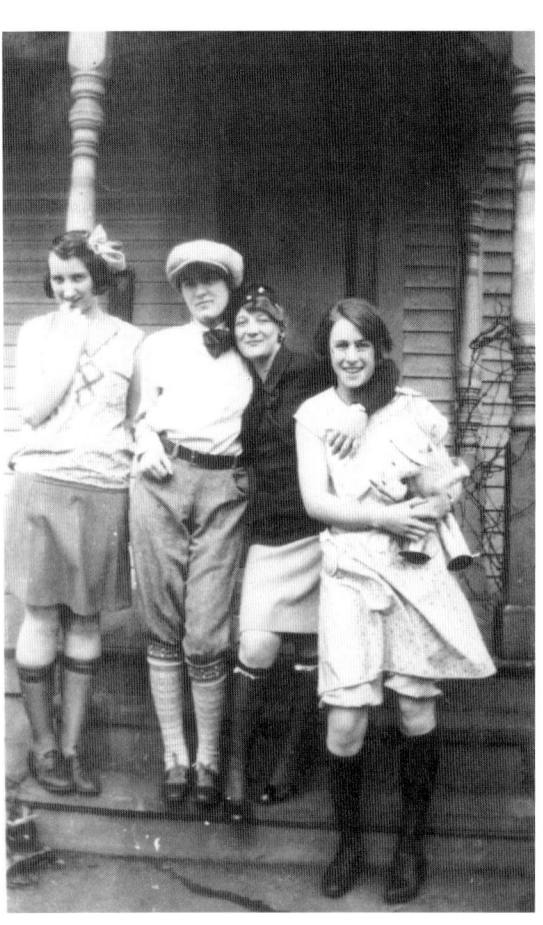

The "kids of Burnside" in 1928

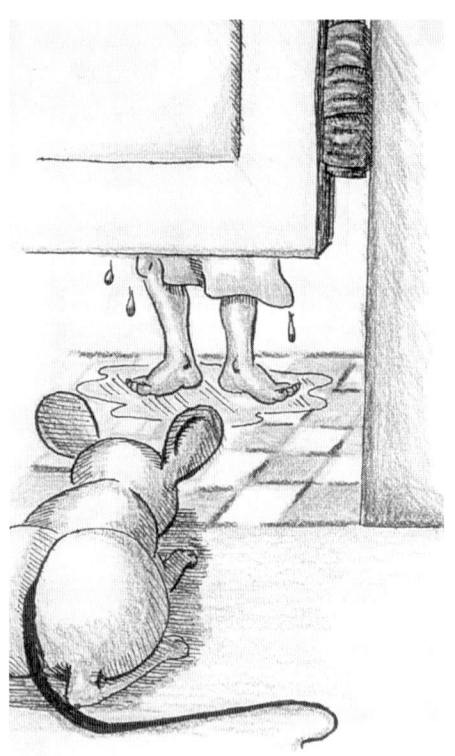

Emma Gutsch Stahnke (1932) drew this sketch of another resident of 222 Earl Street.

5. Thou shalt not ask for late hours for thou shalt not have thy request.
6. Thou shalt not sleep on the roof, lest Miss Parchmann increases her beat.
7. Thou shalt not bathe after ten p.m., lest thou must dry thyself in the dark.
8. Thou shalt not come in through windows, or by means of the basement, lest Miss Larson lies awake.
9. Thou shalt draw thy window shades at Burnside, lest spectators see thee without thy cap.
10. Thou shalt not dissipate at Perry's, lest thou must spend thy hours in widening uniforms.

Helen Sammons Grooms summarized that shared life:

> We were often given the same difficult patient for days on end. We learned a lot about giving real TLC. . . . Of course, we shared joys, too — letters from boy friends, boxes of goodies and candy from home, walks on the bluff on summer evenings. Often, we attended church in a group. Just being teenage girls, giggling over our patients was fun, too.

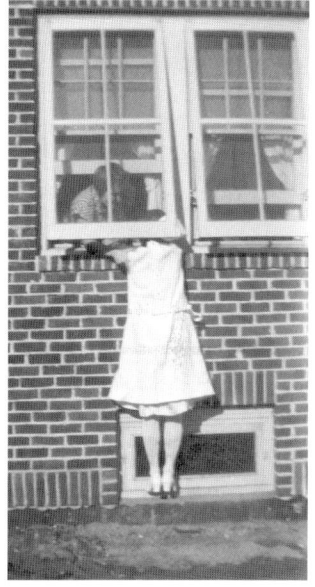

The Cottage, 1927

There were other, more acceptable, outlets for young energy. In 1926, Professor John Jaeger presented Mary Danielson with the idea of beginning a glee club. She readily accepted. He had trained at Ohio Wesleyan Conservatory of Music, was a faculty member at McPhail School of Music, and had directed the glee clubs at Hamline University for sixteen years. The women usually practiced in the basement. It was, Jaeger said, "not exactly conducive to good breathing."

Jaeger became a fixture at Mounds-Midway and the nurses' chorus was an immediate success, garnering numerous awards in its first few years. "There is not a loyal student or alumnus," boasted the *Hospital News* in 1928, "that does not feel a tinge of joy and pride in having a Glee Club of our own to furnish music for Commencement, capping exercises, [and] alumnae meetings."[17]

"Professor Jaeger was small in stature but long on patience," Arita Anderson Malam (1953) remembered. "He had a deep appreciation for good, sacred music and taught us well. This student choir practiced weekly. Then, on pre-scheduled Sunday evenings, we sang in various churches around the Twin Cities. We were in full uniform for these

Chapter Two 55

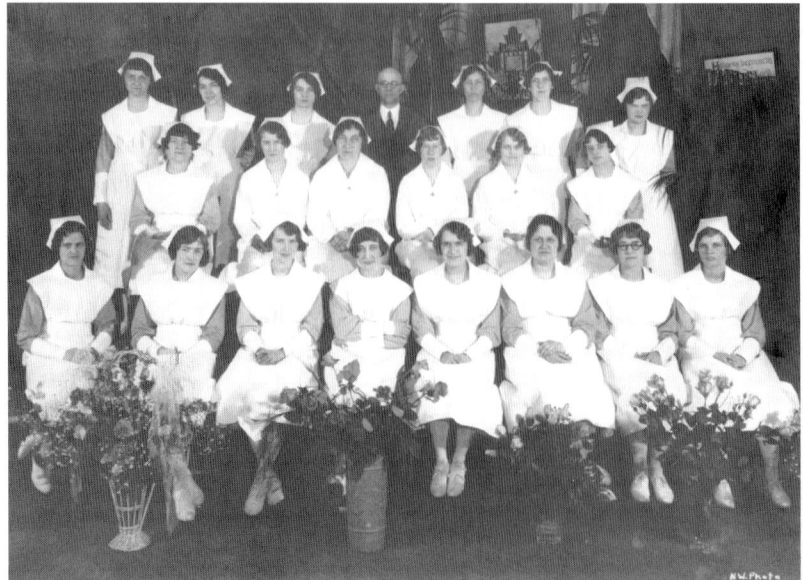

The first Glee Club in 1926. Professor Jaeger stands in the back row.

appearances which usually lasted for about one hour. Interspersed with the music there was opportunity for three or four students to give brief testimonies. At times it seemed that the choir activities were an added demand on our already crowded study and work schedules."

Marjorie Sundin Moor (1940) wrote: "Mr. Jaeger, or 'Prof' as we called him, led the choir through various types of music. Our ministry was to the churches in the area, at graduations, caroling in the halls of the hospital at Christmas time. Once we even ventured as far as Cambridge for a program. The fact that we wore black shoes and stockings (except for the seniors) did not seem to matter."

One early member, Caroline Krueger (1929), emphasized that the glee club was not just a peripheral social gathering, but made them better nurses, writing:

Sing? Why, yes, to be sure
We shall better endure,
If the heart's full of song
All day long.[18]

As Irene Smith said, "I'll never forget the glee club."

The Alumni Association remained active throughout these years and contributed to the students' academic and social life. Every year, the Association bestowed the Kirbach-Dahlby Memorial Scholarship and assisted with learning opportunities for other students by donating library books. On the social calendar, they sponsored the annual Homecoming Tea and the Senior Banquet. As a professional association, they monitored changes in the field of nursing, and, in the early 1940s, began a quarterly newsletter filled with letters from alumni.

At its center, Mounds-Midway was a religious institution, and it began with the type of girl admitted to the school. "One of the fundamental qualifications . . . is that of character," wrote George Earl in 1932. "One who has character for nursing, possesses a soul quality which endows her with a sympathetic understanding of human nature; gives her a keen insight into the needs of hearts and minds; presents a penetrating, alert, and inspiring personality." He added, "This emphasis has been maintained under the regime of our present Superintendent of Nurses."

School records give a glimpse of the denominational background of the students in 1927.

Baptist	82
Lutheran	13
Mission Covenant	4
Christian & Missionary Alliance	2
Evangelical Free	2
Presbyterian	2
Congregational	1
Methodist	1
Protestant	1
Total	108

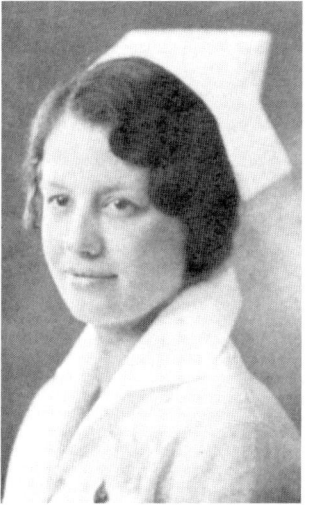

Almyra Eastlund (1931), missionary to Assam, India

Although the numbers varied from year to year, the student body remained predominately Baptist with a significant number of Lutherans.

That core faith was reflected in the daily life of the students. They were required to attend chapel services at 6:30 every morning. The alumni contributed their part as well, with former graduates hosting a bi-monthly Bible study in their homes. Every student took a ten-hour course in the Bible, taught for many years by Rev. E. T. Dahlberg.

There was also a strong missions emphasis, with eight graduates in the field during the relative peaceful years of the 1930s. These included Rosalie Olson, now in Kodiak, Alaska, Margaret Lang, Myrtle Carlson (1929), and Laura Reddig (1933) in Nigeria, and Elna Forsell Avey (1931), Almyra Eastlund Anderson (1931), and Edna Pearson Holm (1929) serving in Assam, India. Back home, the Mission Circle at Mounds-Midway met regularly, held prayer meetings, passed out missionary pamphlets, and collected baskets for needy families in Saint Paul.

World War II

War erupted in Europe in the fall of 1939. Florence Forsyth, living in Vancouver, British Columbia, wrote to the alumni newsletter, lamenting, "This awful war. It is like a bad dream we are again going through. All this misery and grief again in our lives. We don't want America to go to war, but we wish they would speed up the plane factories and get more planes to Britain. Over here, we realize how serious things are, but we wonder if the USA does."[19]

Pearl Harbor brought home the reality of those distant events, and within months, the school and the hospitals were swept up in the national crusade against the Axis powers. Several recent graduates enlisted in the military even before December 7, 1941, including Erla Cranmer (1940), Anna Garbisch (1938), Mary Guderian (1939), Elizabeth Husson (1937), Selma Johnson (1924), Emma Manehr (1916), Dagney Miller (1935), and Mary White (1938). Others joined soon after graduation.

They regularly sent reports back to friends and family, relating the new experiences. Myrtle Nereson Quamen (1939), stationed at Ft. Lewis, Washington, wrote to Mary Danielson:

> Last month, I had my twenty-eight nights of seven p.m. to seven a.m. That was a brutally murderous shift, and I hope that civilian nurses have not had to resort to twelve hours duty. There were four nurses on nights. I had eight wards and averaged 325 patients since the nurse gives all the medications and treatments, I literally ran my legs off. Of course, there are nurses and nurses, but far be it from a Mounds-Midway graduate to consider her book work first and her patients second.

Jeanne Hillis, writing from Walla Walla, Washington, wrote about the transition from student nurse to life in the military: "Our uniforms have arrived, and those of us who have ours ready are now in uniform all the time. I was the first to wear mine . . . and was much embarrassed by all the attraction and comments. There was a possibility I hadn't thought of. When I walked over to the PX and was saluted by two enlisted men. Not having practiced saluting, I gave them a very limp salute in return, and have resolved to learn how." Although Lois Miller thought the uniforms "rather smart looking," she complained that she was "reminded of good old training days when we put on the regulation black shoes and hose again."[20]

As they traveled to distant cities and military bases, they sometimes found reminders of life back at their old school. Margaret Lumsden (1930) related an experience shared by many graduates in far-flung corners of the earth:

> Imagine my surprise at a Red Cross rally in Detroit last year, with 4000 persons present, to have someone touch my arm and say "Hello, Mounds Midway." It was Alberta Jensen, a classmate of mine, whom I had not seen since graduation twelve years before. The greatest surprise was at one of our unit meetings here on the post. When each new member was asked to stand and give her name, who should be there, but Helen Cook, who was an anesthetist at Midway, while I was in training. This is a very small world, and Mounds Midway is well known.[21]

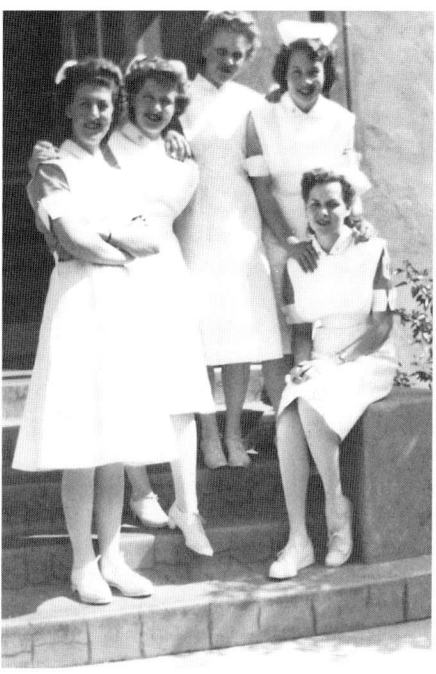

Cadet nurses at Balboa Navy Hospital, San Diego, California. Left to right: M. Nohre, Ardis Williamson Denner, Jeanette Mundheim Adams, Maxine Sigfred Allert, Donna Larson Eddy.

Soon, they would be off to war themselves, seeing service in the Pacific, European, and Mediterranean theaters. Through it all, they carried underlying belief in the war effort. "I shudder to think of what will happen to us if we are taken over by the Japs," wrote Ruth Olan (1927) from Hawaii in 1942. Myrtle Nereson Quamen summed up the typical attitude, writing:

> God is smiling on our type of life, on our ideals, and on our cause. It gives you the strength to believe that we will win this war, and convinces you that all this is worth fighting for. Each time I stand retreat and witness a dress parade, I am more proud to be an American, and I am more proud to be a part of the Army.[22]

Less glamorous, perhaps, but equally challenging and just as important, was the part being played by those nurses who remained at their posts on the home front. As Mary Danielson wrote, "Babies must be borne, surgery performed, and acute illnesses given immediate attention. Civilian health must be maintained and civilian nurses are needed to do it."[23]

Around the hospitals, there were signs of war everywhere. Students

Chapter Two 59

recalled the noise from Holman Field, where work was being done on airplanes. In the middle of the night, its beacon lights would flash across dorm windows. Young men, including many doctors, appeared in uniform, saying goodbye before being shipped out. Soon, there were shortages of doctors, nurses, and supplies. Elese Kerr, president of the Alumni Association, summed up how the war had come home in November 1942:

> Our nation is at war! How often we have heard these very words, but somehow, we didn't grasp their true meaning until we saw the many preparations taking place to protect our homeland — until we heard the bombers flying low to go to the airfields — until we saw the youths, clad in various uniforms on the city streets — until we heard the plea, over the radio, for 'More doctors! More nurses!'[24]

Cadet Nurse Corps

In spite of a nationwide call for nurses, student applications dropped in 1942. "The number of nurses needed by the military forces is gradually increasing," Mary Danielson wrote, "but many other fields had been glamorized to the extent that the nursing profession could not compete." The school sent letters out to Baptist organizations, seeking candidates. Yet, when the American Baptist Missionary Society suggested admitting students from other races, the school responded that it was "not the policy of the school to accept such students." However, Mounds-Midway did receive approval from the U. S. Immigration Service to accept non-quota immigrant students — the school could now accept Canadians.[25]

A dramatic change took place the following year, when Congress passed the Bolton-Bailey Act, funding a major expansion of nurses' training. A school newsletter described the program:

> By entering a school, a student nurse can not only gain a profession without paying the tuition, but she also receives a stipend monthly during her period of training. It also has a strong appeal due to the fact that she feels she is identifying herself with a national emergency, and secures an attractive outdoor uniform. The only requirement is that they remained

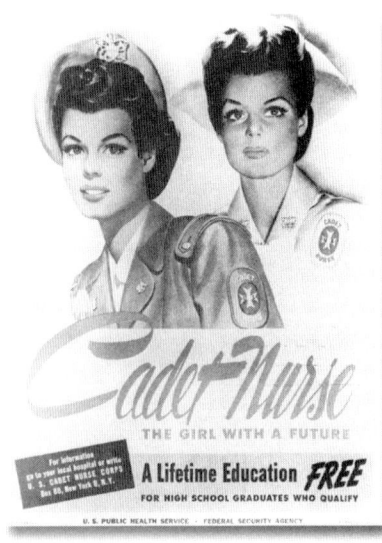

Recruiting poster for the Cadet Nurse Corps.

in nursing for the duration. This need not be military, but may be in federal or any essential civilian nursing service.[26]

Now, for the first time, there was money available for nursing students. The curriculum was accelerated so that all required class work could be completed in thirty months, leaving the last six months of the three-year course for senior cadet experience. This, according to the plan, freed up graduate nurses to serve in the military. Three instructors were added: Ardis Grotey, Marion Bell, and Bessie Youngdahl.

In a newsletter, Miss Danielson described the response: "In our own school, the program is being set in motion. There are fifteen Senior Cadets in the school. Of these, one is doing rural nursing in a northern Minnesota Hospital, three are going to Ancker Hospital for a six-week experience in contagion, and the others are remaining at Mounds-Midway for experience in ward administration and supervision. The purpose of this type of program is to enable the Senior Cadets to assume greater responsibility in that they may take the places of graduate nurses who are needed in the military services."

The school flourished, now flush with money and eager applicants. By the following year, all of the students, except three seniors and two juniors, were Cadet Nurses. Ardis Williamson Denner (1946) remembered, "In the Cadet Nurse program, students took over much of the floor duty and daily care of patients, in addition to a full course load of studies which included pharmacology, anatomy, chemistry, and physiology. The Cadets freed up the graduate nurses to go into the military."

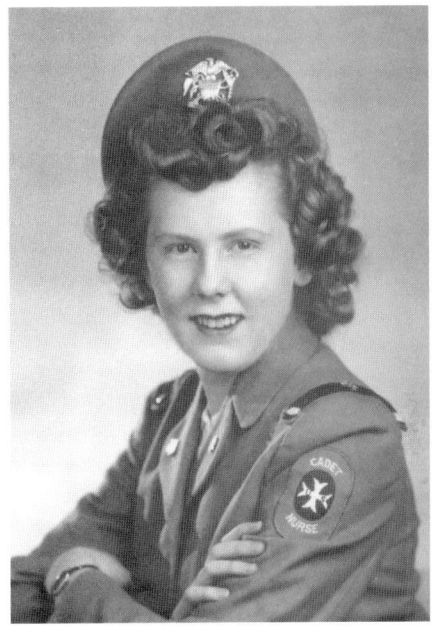

*June Anderson Wallin,
Class of 1947
Cadet Nurse*

There were other benefits, as Bernice Thorson Lemon (1947) recalled: "Our tuition was reimbursed and we got a stipend. We could even buy stamps now! We got to go to movies at serviceman's prices. We could go cheaper by train in uniform and often we would go to the USO stations and watch troop maneuvers. A big thing was to go to a downtown St. Paul hotel's dining room and have a real treat of pecan pie and coffee."

One direct result of the war was the addition of two nurses' homes, funded through the National Defense Housing Act.

At Mounds Park, the nurses' cottage was moved (facing Burns Avenue) to make way for a new dormitory. This new one-story was connected with the basement of 220 Earl Street by a heated tunnel.

A new dorm, later known as Robert Earl Hall, was built in 1945. It is the rectangular building to the left of the main hospital.

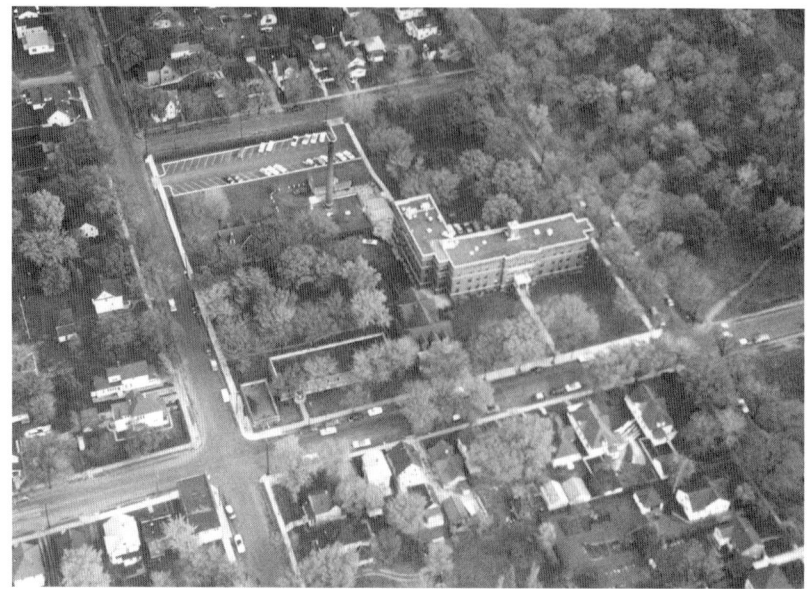

The building, 126 feet long and 44 feet deep, was a full two stories in the back where the ground sloped down. On the first floor there was a reception room, accommodations for a house mother, and thirty-two student nurses. On the ground floor, there was a large classroom, and a new nursing art class and demonstration room, equipped with four demonstration beds. It included such luxuries as offices for the teaching staff, a kitchen for social functions, and a laundry for student nurses' personal use.[27]

At Midway the Federal Works Agency bought a substantial apartment building about half a block from the hospital. It was remodeled and redecorated to accommodate thirty-five student nurses, with one apartment set aside for two graduate supervising nurses. One apartment with kitchenette on the ground floor was used for student nurses as a recreation room. There was also a new classroom, a library, a trunk room, and a laundry for the use of the nurses.[28]

The war apparently loosened the chains of custom as well. Students had always detested the frumpy black shoes and stockings forced on the freshmen and juniors, then tossed in a bonfire as they became seniors ("Do we admit to smoking a cigar that night?" asked Helen Sammons Grooms). On March 1, 1944, all students were allowed to wear white shoes and stockings. Some gathered together on the High Bridge to toss the frumpy black stockings into the Mississippi, with newspaper cameramen recording the momentous event.

Most of Mounds-Midway's 209 Cadet Nurses recall the program

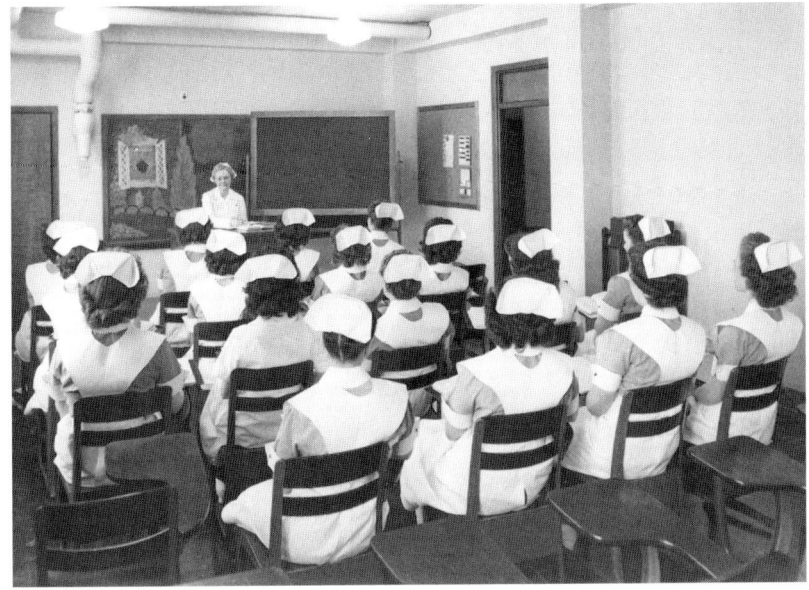

Ruth Gustafson teaches a class, 1942.

fondly. As Jeanne Axelson (1947) wrote, "Many of us, without this opportunity, would never have been nurses." Speaking for all the students who lived through the turbulent war years, she said, "Several of our class have had experiences in veterans and rural hospitals in wards of contagious diseases. Above all we want to be workers together with the great physician, for as that familiar poem reads, to be a nurse is to walk with God, along the paths that our master trod. The purpose of our service is that we may lead the restless into rest, the wounded into healing, the wearied home, and the lost back again to the heart of God."

The Post–War Years

The Cadet Corps ended shortly after the surrender of Japan in August 1945, although those already in the program would continue to receive financial aid. Without these financial incentives, though, new applications dropped dramatically. No class was admitted in February 1946. A class of thirty-four entered in August 1946, but, in February 1947, only thirteen students were admitted. In August 1947, thirty-two students began training.[29]

The war years, though, left a new sense of professional pride. Hours were eased slightly, based on the recommendation of the Board of Examiners of Nurses. During the probationary period, students could have ten hours of clinical practice each week, but were given every other weekend off and every other Friday afternoon. For the other students, it was a forty-eight hour a week schedule — including class work — with one full day off each week and a half-day on holidays. Ten weeks of vacation were granted during the three years.

The new professionalism translated into several new initiatives in the curriculum. The "Supervised Clinical Experience," a term used for the first time in the 1947 bulletin of the school, included:

Preclinical Term	20 weeks	Mounds Park
Medical service	24 weeks	Mounds Park
Surgical Service	24 weeks	Midway Hospital
Diet Therapy	6 weeks	Midway Hospital
Operating Room	8 weeks	Midway Hospital
Obstetrical Service	14 weeks	Midway Hospital
Emergency and Outpatient	3 weeks	Midway or Mounds
Neuropsychiatry	18 weeks	Mounds Park
Pediatrics	13 weeks	Children's Hospital
Communicable Service	6 weeks	Ancker Hospital
Assignments or electives	10 weeks	Midway or Mounds

Among the most notable changes was an affiliation with Ancker Hospital in communicable diseases, begun in 1946. "What a lot of different experiences we have," wrote one student about this new clinical experience. "Have you seen the enlarged Stenson's duct on a mumps patient? Can you distinguish between the macular, papular, vesicular, and scab stages in chicken pox? are you familiar with the grayish membrane in the throat of a diptheria patient?"[30]

Among the other clinical rotations, obstetrics was always lively, especially in the early post-war years as the first wave of the baby boom hit. As a senior, Edna Carlson Hughes (1947) was working an evening shift when the unexpected happened. She wrote, "This lady was in labor. the doctor had checked her not too long before, and all seemed to be going nicely when, lo and behold, she felt constrained to push. I called the supervisor and went to the patient's bedside. Here comes one of the cutest babies you ever saw. the supervisor came rushing in and I was holding a baby up by its feet."

Life of a Student Nurse after the War

Bernice Thorson Lemon (1947): "What do I remember about February 1944? It was a snowy Minnesota day and my father drove Lylah Runningen and me the 150 miles from Houston to St. Paul. All of

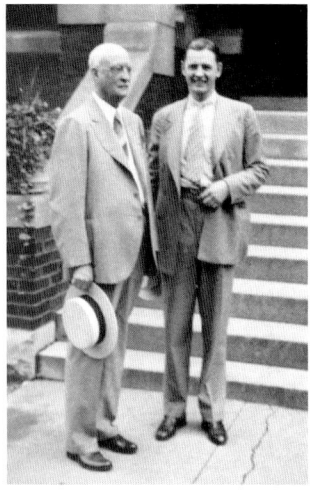

Dr. Robert Earl and his son, John, in 1942, shortly before John entered military service.

The Doctors

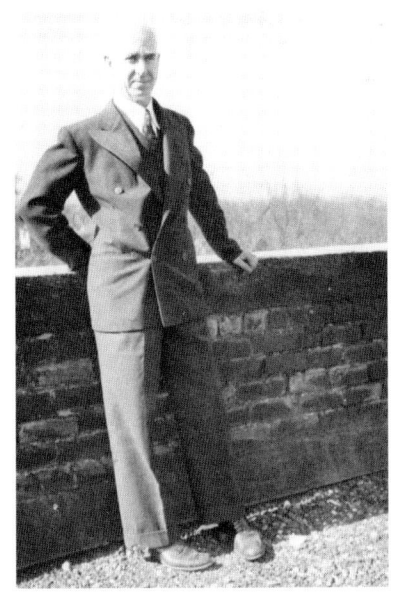

Dr. Archibald Leitch

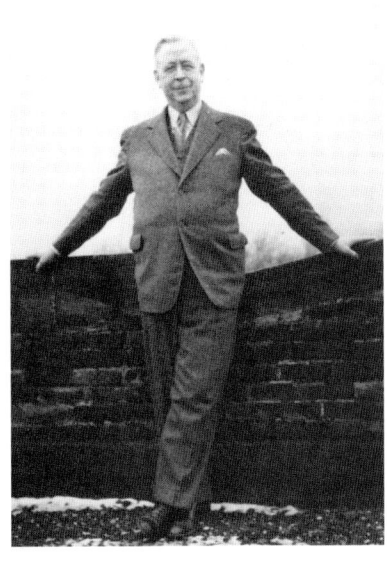

Dr. Robert Burns

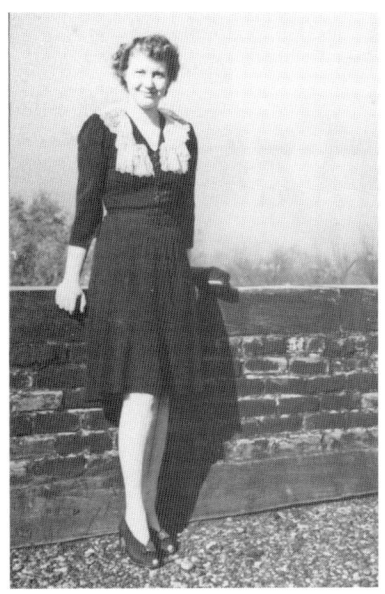

Dr. Eva Ostergren Larson

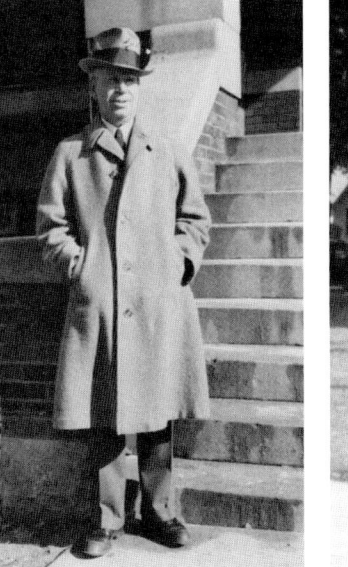

Dr. Gilbert Kvitrud

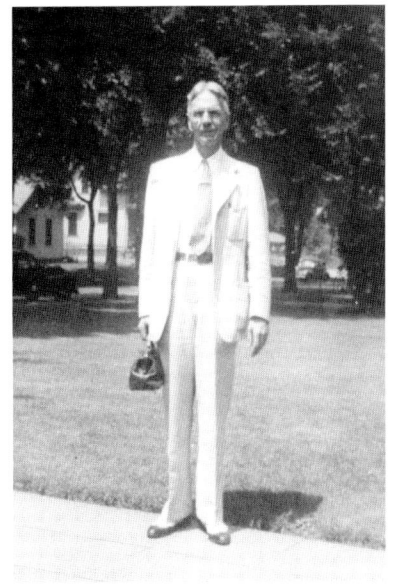

Dr. E. Hammes

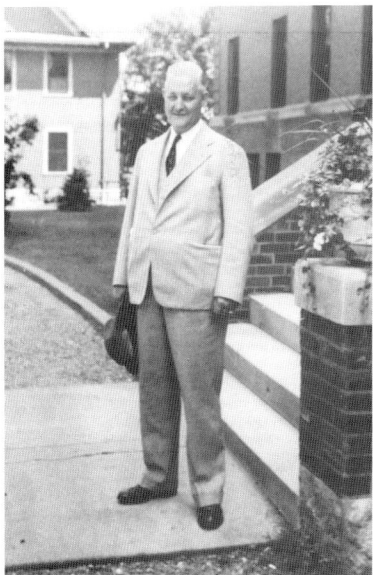

Dr. Edward W. Ostergren

Chapter Two

Social Life

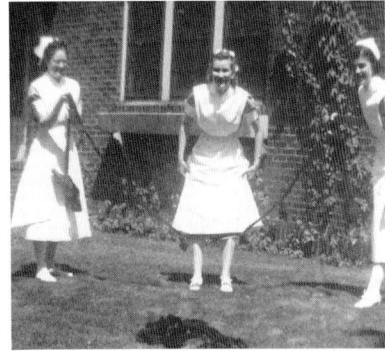

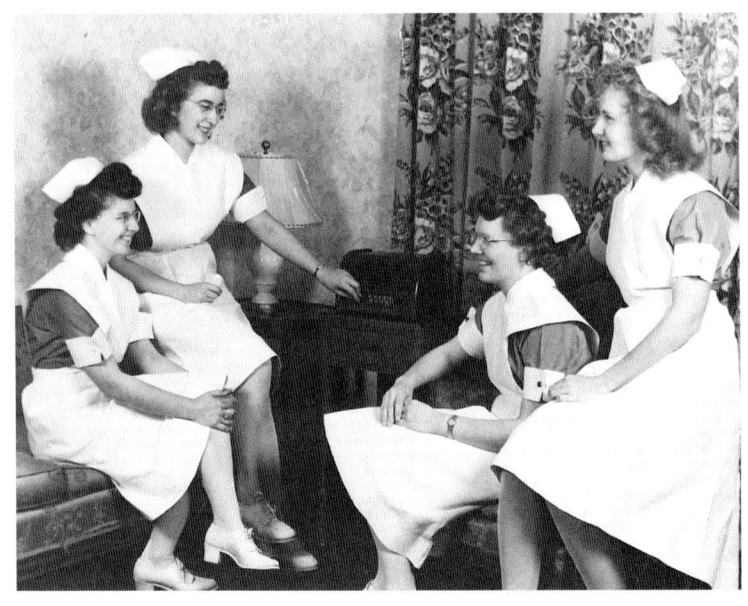

Above left: Getting rid of the dreaded black stockings. Above right: Enjoying the new radio at Robert Earl Hall: Grace Siebel (1949), Donna Treleaven (1949), Marie Pegors (1948), Virginia Lennberg (1948)

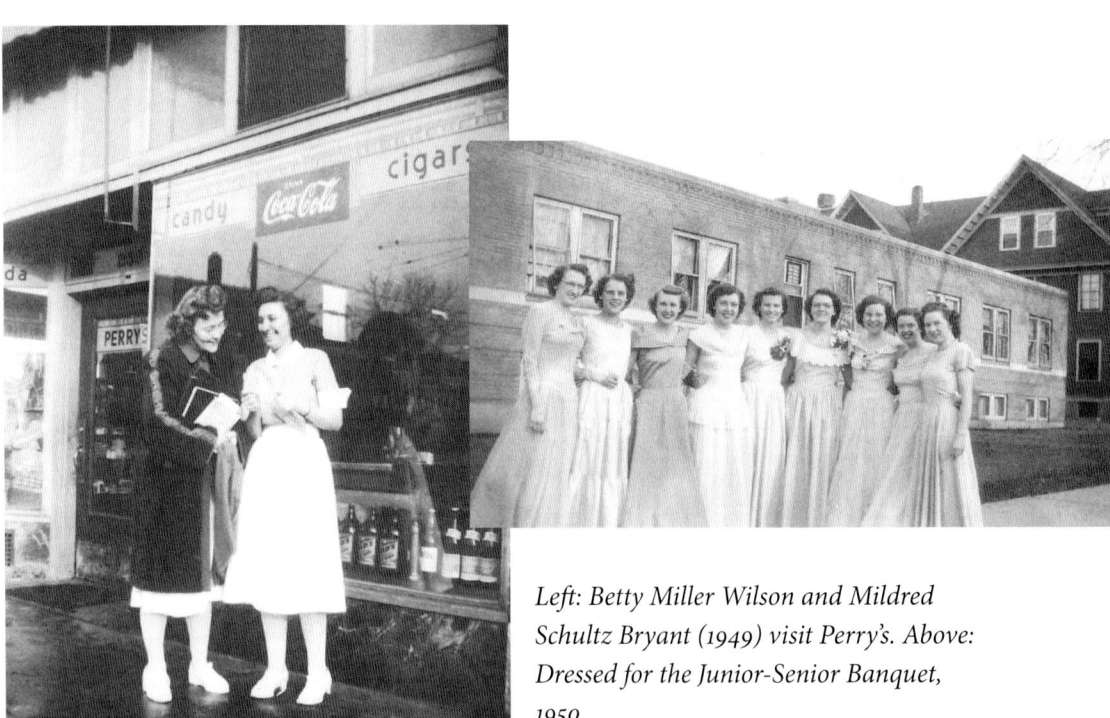

Left: Betty Miller Wilson and Mildred Schultz Bryant (1949) visit Perry's. Above: Dressed for the Junior-Senior Banquet, 1950.

my earthly belongings were in one trunk. We lived at Burnside dormitory with five students and two instructors. I was so homesick that I cried. Not wanting Miss Nelson or Miss Garnett to see me, I hid in a closet."

Life in the dorm could be an adventure. "It wasn't exactly the Waldorf-Astoria," said Janet Valine Larson (1951) about the dorms. "I remember my arrival at Mounds Park, third floor, old dorm. There was one bathroom on each floor. Everyone shared one telephone located in the hallway on second floor." Of course, "home" would be in different places over the course of three years. "Many of us moved our belongings by streetcar to Midway or Children's Hospital," Donna Larson Eddy (1946) remembered. "We owned an orange crate that was a cupboard for our books that could then be taken along whenever we moved. During our second year, some of us lived in a section of the first-floor patient rooms used for a dormitory."

As the students worked and studied, there were many other people who touched their lives every day. Betty Bonin, sometimes known as "Elevator Betty", took a job as elevator operator at Mounds Park in 1943. As the years went on, she gained more responsibility, often assisting patients as they moved between floors. In 1957, she returned to school, then moved to the Medical Records Department, working with Ebba Peterson. She remained at Mounds until 1986.

Or there was Bill Carlson, the hospital's chief engineer. He started at Mounds Park in 1917 as an elevator boy, then, in 1919, he was hired to work on the crew shoveling coal for the boilers. In his spare time, he was occasionally asked to move patients or help out in the kitchen. Carlson stayed on the job for more than fifty years.

Vernon Sommerdorf received his first introduction to Mounds-Midway through his cousin, Orva Ewald, a student at the school in 1937. She often brought her friends over to the house, and "as a high school junior," he wrote, "I found these 'older women' to be quite sophisticated and even a bit glamorous." After World War II, he began pre-med studies at the University of Minnesota and worked part-time as a male nurse at Mounds Park. "I do remember getting in trouble with Violet Nelson on one occasion," Dr. Sommerdorf admitted. "She did not like the tradition of tearing the student uniforms on the last day they were worn and when she found out that I had participated in this ritual, she became quite upset."

Then there was Jewel—fondly called "our diamond in the rough." The 1949 *Pre-RN* described her as "an unforgettable character."

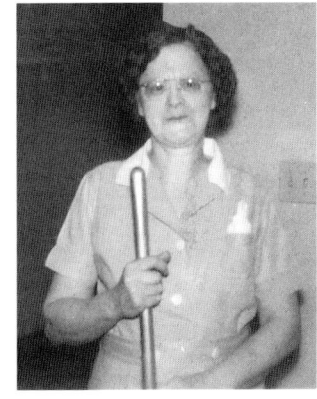

Jewel

Chapter Two 67

Clickety-clack, clickety-clop. Swish, swish, bang bang, plop. Then a rasping voice says cheerily, "Good morning, girls. Oh, are you sleeping?" wearily . . . you wonder, what is it? An earthquake? A hurricane? Cautiously, you open your eyes only to behold clouds of dust billowing around them. . . . Suddenly, you feel a tug underneath you and zoom! "This is laundry day. You know, girls, you can't sleep all day!" As the door opens, you hear, "The sheets have to be counted!"

Students also learned from quiet ministries, like Mr. Kampher's, whose daughter, Dorothy Kampher Fritz, graduated from the school in 1928. After his wife died at Mounds—to show his thanks for the care that she received in her last days—he provided transportation. Lauralie Nelson Robertson, (1950) said, "He was a widower and was a big help to us taking us to church, Sunday afternoon rides, and helping us to move our stuff from one hospital to the other." Others remember that he often brought tomatoes or apples, treasured as evening snacks. When asked why he did it, he answered, "This is one bit of missionary work that I can do and I am so happy that I can do it."

"All work and no play makes Jill a dull girl," declared students Mabel Derkson (1950) and Alice Stenstrom (1951) in an article in the *American Journal of Nursing*. They provided a summary of social calendar of a Mounds-Midway girl in the late forties, including special events centered around the holidays, the monthly birthday teas, and occasional dramas or skits. Then, for physical outlets, there were highly competitive ping pong matches and the legendary bed-making contest of 1949.[31]

One of the longstanding traditions was that of "Big Sister-Little Sister," as described in the article: "One of the older students, without revealing her identity, acts as a big sister to the new student with encouraging letters and small gifts. The climax is reached with a special party near the end of the preliminary period, at which the identity is revealed." Many graduates, forty years later, still keep in touch with their old big or little sisters.

There were boyfriends, although many were in the military and so remained only a framed photograph or well-worn letter to the students. The girls received careful supervision. Alice Hoglund McKee (1948) remembered one cold wintry night when she had a late pass. Her fiancee had driven sixty-five miles to see her. McKee wrote, "We had gone to the social room in the dormitory at Midway Hospital

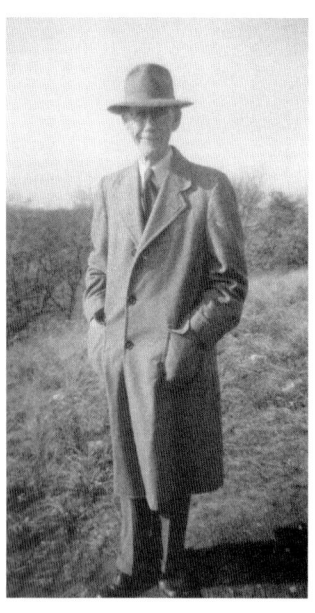

Charles Kampher

Mrs. Chase and friends

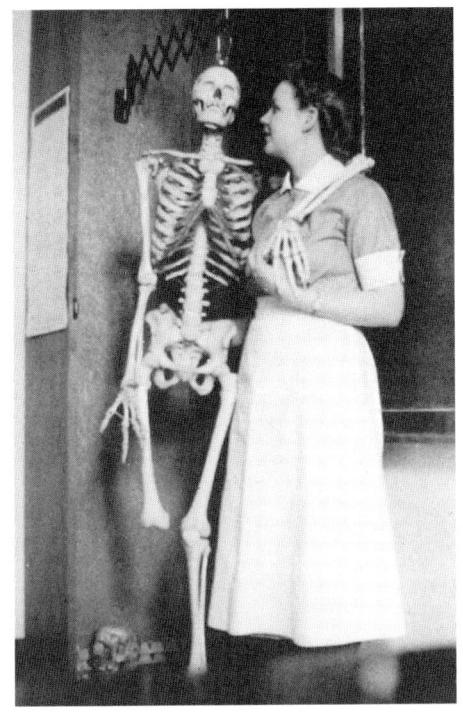

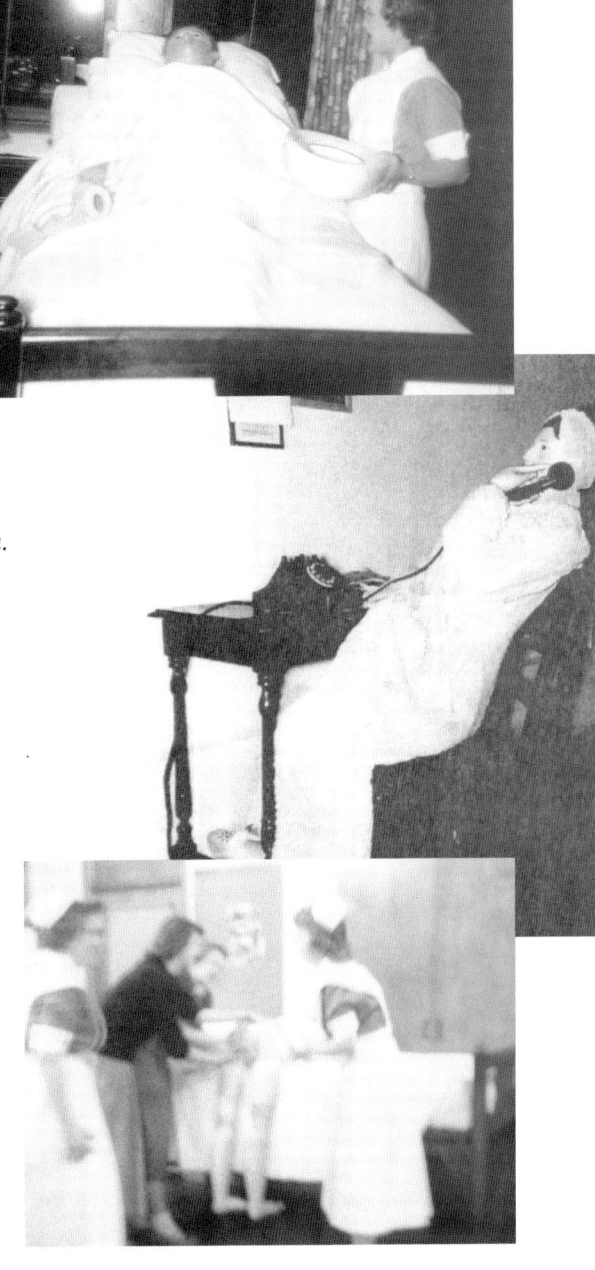

Upper left: Donna Larson Eddy (1946).
Upper right: Mrs. Chase needs to use the bedpan.
Right: Mrs. Chase on the phone.
Lower right: Mrs. Chase receives an exam.
Below: Violet Nelson, Backwards Day party.

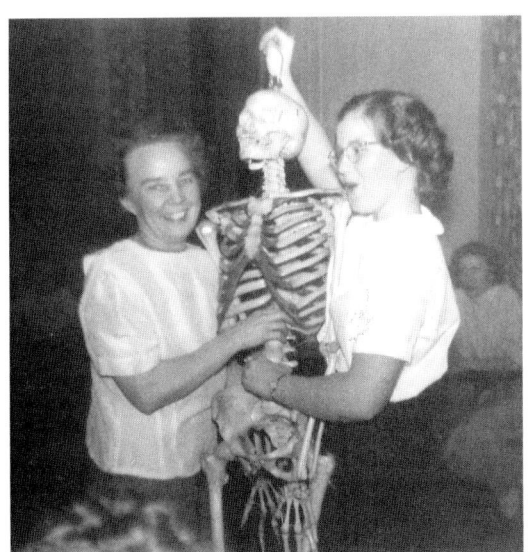

Chapter Two 69

due to the cold outdoors. Miss Grandin found us there and informed us that I was to be in my room after the ten p.m. curfew. My fiancee asked her if it would have been better for us to have sat outdoors in the car in the cold. I was put on restriction for two weeks because he had been impertinent to her." Of course, McKee had the last laugh, secretly marrying months before graduation.

The school also organized its first Student Association in 1948, bringing all the activities under one umbrella organization. Members also represented Mounds-Midway in the new Minnesota Student Nurses Association.

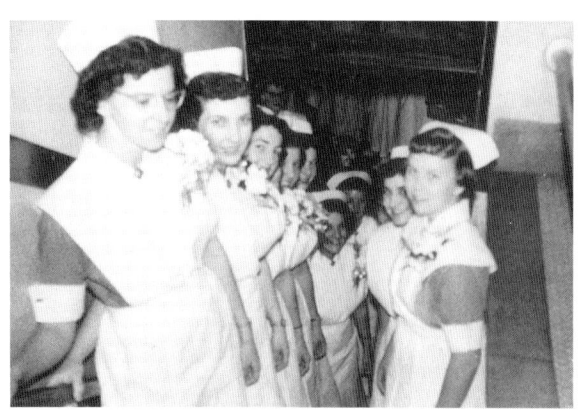

Students were presented gardenias on capping day.

Spiritual activities were important amidst a busy schedule, and a new organization, Intervarsity Christian Fellowship, promoted such activities as daily prayer meetings, weekly Bible study classes, and monthly devotional programs as well as missionary interests both at home and abroad. Others students recall the young people's rallies in Saint Paul with a songleader named Cliff Barrows. Afterwards, he often drove student nurses home. "And he was such a good-looking guy," added June Anderson Wallin (1947).

Reflecting on the impact of those years, Stella Samuelson Pearson (1946) wrote, "I felt very close to God when we were privileged to hear the scripture read, hear it discussed a little, and closed with a word of prayer." Mary Jenkins Olson (1945) concurred: "To this day, I am grateful for the Christian atmosphere in the hospitals and school. The early morning chapel services are held in fond memories, especially the singing of 'Blest Be the Tie' on the last day of each student. Some Christian fellow students, with whom I still have close friendships, helped encourage me in faith."

Janet Valine Larson (1951) remembered graduation, "The service was at the First Baptist Church in downtown St. Paul. At the closing of the service, Professor Jaeger led one nurses' chorus singing a hymn, 'O Jesus, I Have Promised to Serve Thee to the End.' I was honored to sing one stanza of this hymn as a solo with the chorus. And it has always been my prayer."

An era was coming to an end. In 1948, Dr. Robert Earl died. Although slowed by a heart attack a decade earlier, he remained active and had been at his office the day before his death. Accolades poured in from across the nation, but none more touching than the one given by his brother, who wrote, "He was a man of dignity, and yet of marked graciousness, a man of ability and yet very humble, a man given to justice with marked sincerity and sympathy." The new dormitory at Mounds Park was named in his honor.[32]

At the same time, Mary Danielson began to suffer a series of medical problems, primarily related to her heart, and spent three months in the hospital. Through war and peace, depression and boom, the two had led Mounds-Midway School of Nursing, but now the winds of change were in the air.

Endnotes

[1] "A living monument for the future," *Northwestern Baptist Hospital Association* (1937).

[2] "Midway District Grows Fast," *Hospital News*, 1 (1928), 1.

[3] Falsum Russell, "Midway Hospital Builder Will Quit After 42 Years," *St. Paul Sunday Pioneer Press*, 23 December 1968.

[4] "Tributes to Miss Gustafson," *Mounds-Midway News Letter*, 12 (May 1952), 1.

[5] "A living monument for the future," *Northwestern Baptist Hospital Association* (1937).

[6] *School Annual Report, Mounds Midway School of Nursing*, 1936.

[7] Gary Phelps, "A National Epidemic Launches Blue Cross and Blue Shield," *Ramsey County History*, 20 (1985), 3-15.

[8] Isabel Stewart, "Trends in Nursing Education," *American Journal of Nursing*, 31 (May 1931), 601-611.

[9] *Nursing Schools — Today and Tomorrow*, 84

[10] *School Annual Report, Mounds-Midway School of Nursing* (1936).

[11] *Mounds-Midway School of Nursing Alumni Newsletter* (February 1997), 2.

[12] *Information Bulletin, Mounds-Midway School of Nursing* (1938), 13.

[13] Gladys Thorson Newman, *Natalie* (Fletcher, OH: Cam-Tech Publishing, 2001), 61-62.

[14] *Mounds-Midway Nurses Alumnae Association Bulletin* (May 1941), 36.

[15] Minutes, Training School Administrative Committee, 1940, quoted in Espelien, 33.

[16] "Capping exercises," *Mounds Midway News Letter* (Fall 1928).

[17] Carole Nelson, "Retired musician isn't very retiring," *St. Paul Pioneer Press*, 15 February 1969.

[18] "The Nurses' Glee Club," *Hospital News*, 1 (1928), 8.

[19] *Mounds-Midway News Letter* (November 1941).

20. Letters from Alumnae Members, *Mounds-Midway News Letter*, III (April 1943) 5-6.
21. Letters from Alumnae Members, *Mounds-Midway News Letter*, IV (November 1943) 5.
22. Letters from Alumnae Members, *Mounds-Midway News Letter*, III (April 1943) 3-4.
23. Letters from Alumnae Members, *Mounds-Midway News Letter*, V (April 1944) 1.
24. "War! Our Nation is at War," *Mounds-Midway News Letter* (November 1942), 1.
25. Training School Administrative Committee, 1942, quoted in Espelien, 36.
26. Letters from Alumnae Members, *Mounds-Midway News Letter*, IV (November 1943), 2.
27. "Two New Nurses' Homes," *Mounds-Midway News Letter*, V (April 1944) 3.
28. Letter from Robert Earl, *Mounds-Midway News Letter*, VI (November 1944), 1.
29. "Has Mounds-Midway Kept Its Ideals?" *Mounds-Midway News Letter*, 12 (November 1947), 1.
30. *Pre-RN* (May 1949), 6.
31. Mabel Derkson and Alice Stenstrom, "One School's Social Program: These students team up for happy living," *American Journal of Nursing*, 49 (December 1949).
32. *Mounds-Midway News Letter*, 13 (May 1948), 2.

CHAPTER THREE
A Sisterhood

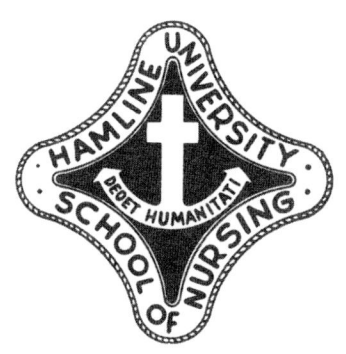

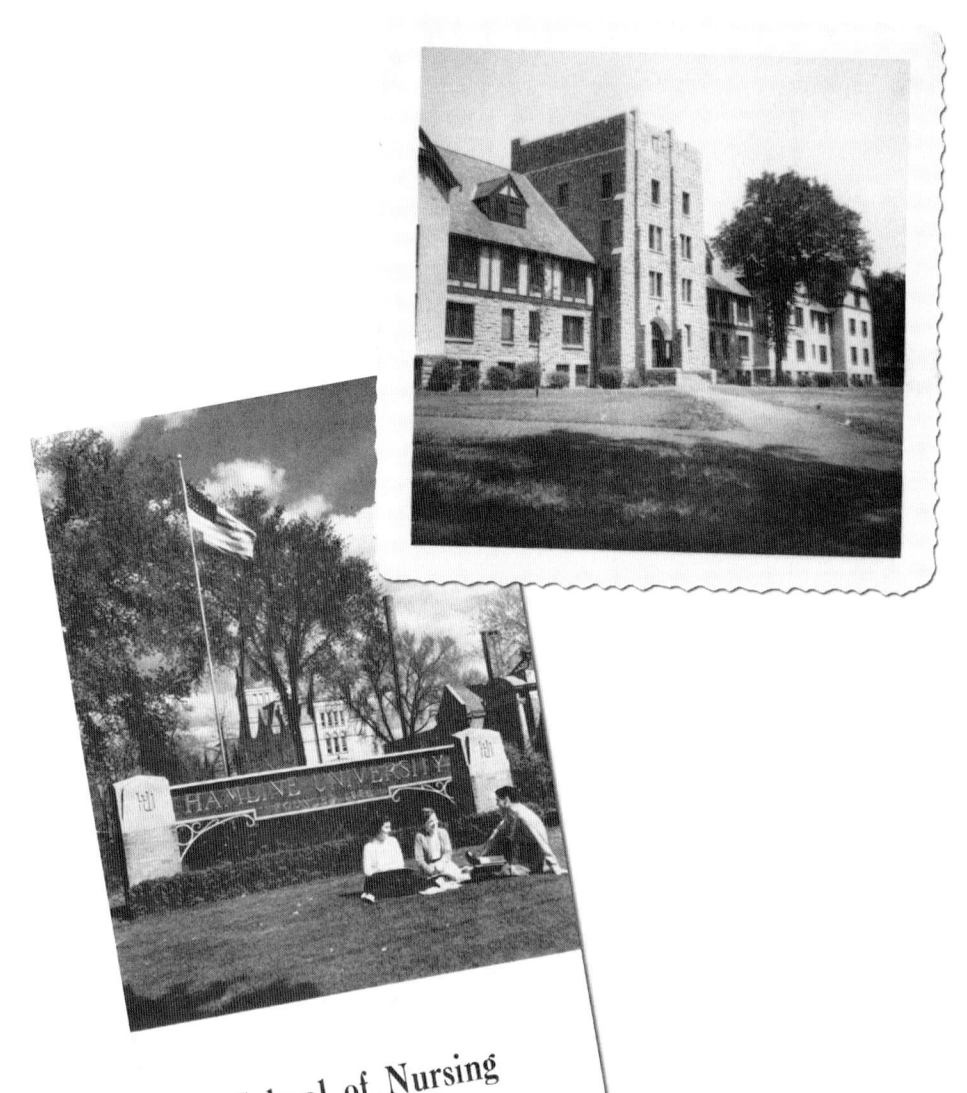

*T*HE SUDDEN INFLUX OF students and money during the war years, followed by several years of quiet change, altered the nursing profession. After a shortage of students in the years following the war, enrollments began to grow again, aided by tremendous growth in hospital construction and the first impact of the "Baby Boom". To meet the demand, a new licensing program, Practical Nursing, spread across the country, offering a quick route into nursing.

By 1949, Mounds-Midway could look back over a highly successful decade. Enrollment had crept back up to pre-Cadet Corps levels and a new Midway dorm at 425 Aldine was on the drawing boards. Faculty tenure remained fairly stable, and the school hired its first full-time librarian that year. In addition, a new affiliation in communicable diseases began with Ancker Hospital, broadening the opportunity for education. Measured by professional standards, the quality of the training was evidenced by the fact that fewer than three percent of its graduates failed the state board examinations in the 1940s. Finally, Mounds-Midway was one of the first three schools in the Twin Cities to have a National League for Nursing accreditation visit before it was required.[1]

The 1949 report of the National Committee for the Improvement of Nursing Services rated Mounds-Midway in the top quartile nationally for the quality of the teaching staff, and in the second quartile for its clinical and library facilities. Overall, that placed the school in the fifty to seventy-five percent range nationally.

A series of national trends, however, led to a very dramatic change at Mounds-Midway. In 1948, Esther Lucille Brown, on behalf of the Russell Sage Foundation, published a cogent analysis of nursing education in the report, *Nursing for the Future*. She lamented, "Many thoughtful persons are beginning to wonder why young women in any large numbers would want to enter nursing as practiced, or schools of nursing as operated today."[2]

Dr. Brown's recommendations revolutionized nursing education in the next decade. Brown critiqued the diploma school system, and recommended that "effort be directed to building basic schools of nursing in universities and colleges, that are sound in organizational and financial structure, adequate facilities and faculty, and well distributed to serve the needs of the entire country." She also recommended that a number of small schools close because of a poor performance record.

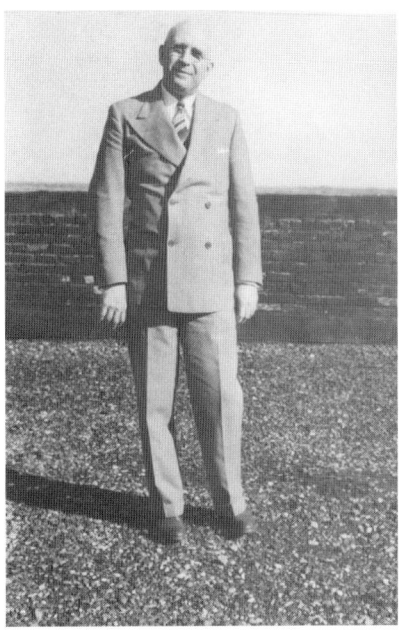

Following the death of his brother, Robert, Dr. George Earl took an increasingly important leadership role in the Northwestern Baptist Hospital Association.

Chapter Three 75

In the interim, the hospital-related schools would need to continue to insure a steady flow of personnel into nursing. However, they needed to be upgraded with better resources for libraries, laboratories, and other physical facilities.

The National League of Nursing Education quickly adopted Brown's recommendations, urging that hospital schools, "give early consideration to the transfer of control and administration to educational institutions."

In other corners, the reaction was swift and negative. As one article asked, "Are nurses getting too much education?" The president of the American Hospital Association, Graham Davis, complained that the Brown report ignored economic reality and threatened to turn the profession into "trade unionism."[3] A new organization, the National Organization of Hospital Schools of Nursing, warned that, "Confusion, discouragement, and even despair exist among nurses, physicians, and hospital administrators. . . .The described conditions burnish fertile fields for the seeds of ideologies, contrary to Americanism." Indeed, because accreditation and the college nursing movement relied upon federal subsidies, and therefore federal control, it would "aid and abet the enemies of free enterprise and freedom."[4]

To the school's credit, the Brown Report quickly had an immediate impact, convincing Mary Danielson that the school of nursing needed to affiliate with a university or college. The 1949 National Committee review, in fact, had given Mounds-Midway a "26-50%" rating in curriculum, based primarily on its weak science program. Always proudly professional, she knew that collegiate affiliation would help the school meet the new goals. In this, she received the full support of Dr. George Earl to explore possibilities. Annette Grandin recalled, "Dr. Earl was a great supporter for the school and took great pride in it and encouraged us to grow and make changes with the recommendations of the National League of Nursing."

The idea was not new. Indeed, a decade earlier, the school seriously considered an affiliation with Bethel Junior College—a school with historic and denominational ties—for science courses. Mary Danielson was hopeful for an agreement, reporting to the state nursing board:

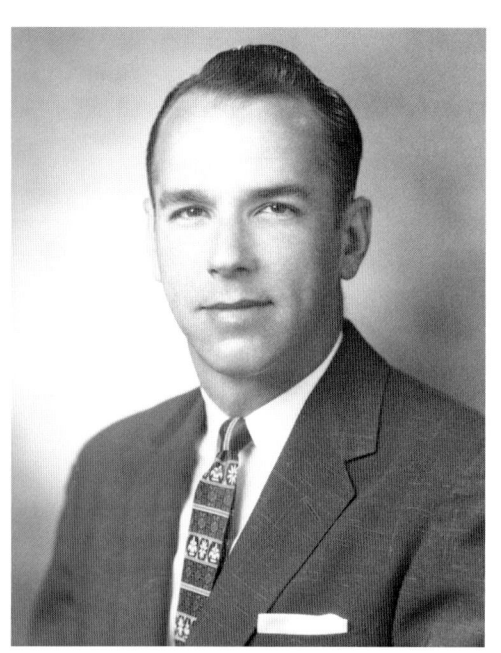

L. Melvin Conley, executive director of the Baptist Hospital Fund.

> A cooperative program with Bethel Junior College is being planned where academic work can be given to the students who are interested before they enter the School of Nursing. This arrangement will be an incentive, especially to nurses who desire to enter the field of education, because with two years of junior college and three years of training the nurse may enter the University of Minnesota or some other senior college for three quarters, or at the most one year, and receive the degree of B.S. This will also help to give us better material for staff appointments.[5]

In the end, final agreement was never reached, but Danielson, who strongly supported a college affiliation, continued to explore other possibilities over the next decade. These included discussions with Bethel College, Hamline University, and Macalester College.

Following the publication of the Brown report and the National League for Nursing recommendations in 1948, the school board decided that the time was ripe for action. Approached again, Bethel held back, wary of taking on additional responsibilities in the midst of its own period of growth. In the fall of that year, Dr. Earl told the state nursing board that Hamline University "seems to be the institution they will approach." Helen Schwartz, that organization's executive secretary, also noted Dr. Earl's belief that Mary Danielson wanted to retire. Negotiations apparently moved rapidly, because by February 1949, a tentative agreement had been reached.[6]

Founded in 1854, Hamline University is Minnesota's oldest university and was named in honor of Leonidas Hamline, a bishop of the

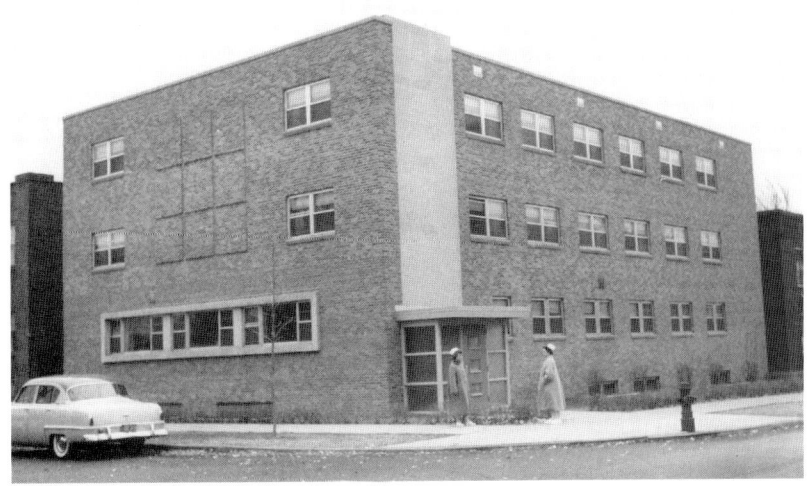

The new Midway dormitory at 425 Aldine Street.

Methodist Church whose interest in the frontier led him to donate funds toward the building of an institution of higher learning in what was then the Territory of Minnesota. From the beginning, it was a coeducational institution — a rarity in nineteenth century America. In 1880, the school moved to the Midway district in Saint Paul, where it grew into a well-respected private institution of higher education.

In 1940, Hamline University and Asbury Methodist Hospital of Minneapolis established the Hamline-Asbury School of Nursing, offering a five-year program (later a four-year) leading to the degree of bachelor of science in nursing. In taking this step, Hamline joined the growing trend in the country to provide academic training for women preparing for careers in nursing. When the older Mounds-Midway School of Nursing approached its board with a request for affiliation, all the pieces were in place.

The prospect, although long discussed, was not without its doubts. After twenty-five years as director, Miss Danielson expressed mixed feelings, as Schwartz reported, "[She] is deeply concerned about Hamline University and Mounds-Midway planning. She seems unwilling to take a leadership role in [it], wants very much to resign because of her health. She seems both eager to have proceedings, yet also reluctant for plans to move ahead and quite obviously feels promotional schemes are going too rapid[ly]. Miss Danielson fears a serious drop in enrollment if this goes ahead."[7]

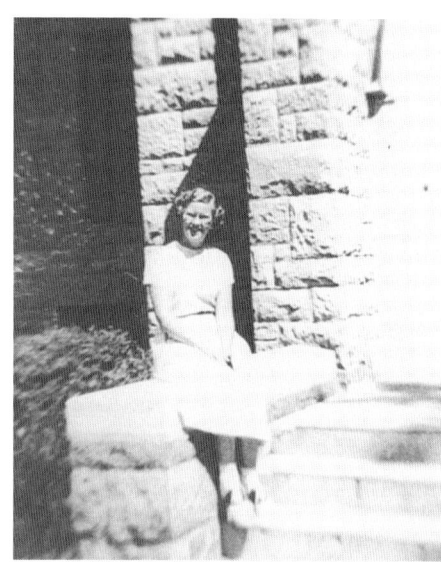

Jeanette Kuhl (1952) on the steps of Manor House, Hamline University, July 1949

There were other concerns as well, particularly because Hamline University was a traditional Methodist school, while Mounds-Midway remained linked to Baptist churches, a major source of financial support. One report said that, "There has been some criticism from the Church Association of closing the school as this has been the only school of nursing under Baptist church denomination in this northwest central area."[8]

On May 31, 1949, a merger between the Mounds-Midway School of Nursing and Hamline University was announced by Hurst R. Anderson, the president of the University. He stated that the new school would be the largest nursing school under church auspices in Minnesota, uniting the Baptist and Methodist communions in a program to meet the need for nurses educated under religious direction. The Hamline School of Nursing now consisted of three divisions: Mounds-Midway Hospital and Asbury Hospital, both diploma programs, and a four-year baccalaureate program.[9]

This began a three-year transition, as students already in the program — the last class being admitted to Mounds-Midway in February 1949 — continued on the same path toward their nursing diploma. Because the move was so rapid, there was inadequate opportunity to fully integrate the next class. This led to a single "experimental" class that graduated in 1952. These students attended Hamline University for a twelve-week course beginning in June 1949, with Mounds-Midway paying for tuition, books, room, and board. One member of the class remembered, "They decided all of a sudden that we should enter in June. I was home, mowing the lawn when Miss Danielson called and said, 'Can you come next week?' I had two jobs. I said, can I think about it? She said, 'We need to know now.' So I put my hand over the phone and asked my parents and they said, go!"

For this class, much remained unchanged after that first summer, including the uniform and cap. It was the last class to have Mary Danielson as director.

For subsequent classes, though, the merger brought more significant changes, beginning at the top. Under Hamline, decisions were made by a coordinating committee, with Mounds-Midway typically represented by Dr. George Earl, Melvin Conley, and Ann Friedsburg. Since his brother's death, George had become the most influential spokesperson for the two hospitals.

Dr. Earl was joined now by Conley, a talented manager who began work as business administrator in 1946, then was appointed executive director of the Baptist Hospital Fund in 1953. After the Northwestern Baptist Hospital Association was placed in receivership in 1933, the BHF was organized as a distinct and separate organization to raise funds for the School of Nursing and provide assistance to the receiver. This arrangement remained in place until 1956, when final payment was made on all receivership claims. This led to the merger of the Northwestern Baptist Hospital Association and Baptist Hospital Fund under the latter name.[10]

Management of the school of nursing shifted from hospital control to the control by an institution of higher education, including a new director after more than two decades of leadership by Mary Danielson. Alice Brethorst had taken the post as dean at the Hamline-Asbury School of Nursing in 1945. She seemed well-suited to lead the new nursing school. Well-educated, she received her R.N. in 1907 from Asbury Hospital School of Nursing. She attended Northwestern College and served as a missionary in China for many years. Returning to the

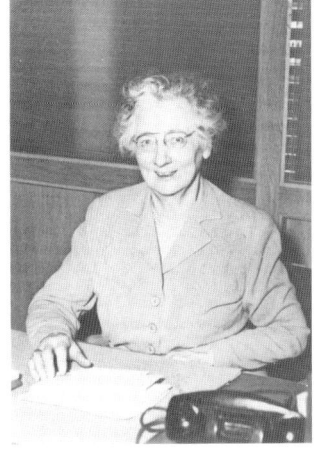

Dr. Alice Brethorst

States, she earned a B.A. in 1922, a M.A. in 1923, and a Ph.D. from the University of Washington in 1931.

The transition took place over the next three years, but when the last class graduated, on November 27, 1952, the Mounds-Midway School of Nursing officially closed.[11]

The merger resulted in changes both large and small. Hamline University hired and paid the faculty. Three educational coordinators, reporting directly to the dean, were named: Ruth Gustafson, Mounds Park Hospital; Annette Grandin, Midway Hospital; and Doris Yokie, Asbury Hospital. Among the most noticeable differences in the new regime was the uniform. The basic dress was light blue, with a white bib — high in front with straps crossing in the back — and a white apron. Students' names were also on their bibs. The cap was patterned after the Asbury School of Nursing, with hemstitching across the band and buttoned in the back with a small pearl button. Seniors wore a black velvet stripe on the right corner of the cap. Still, a student insisted, "Inside, they are still the same warm-hearted Mounds-Midway kids."[12]

Conforming to new national guidelines, hours also changed. All students at Midway and Mounds Park Hospital, were placed on a forty-hour week, including class and clinical practice and now received a four-week vacation each year.

Dr. Brethorst had accepted the additional responsibility of directing a much larger program, with a new division, three campuses, and some 300 students. Given different institutional priorities and distinct long-standing cultures, the merger would prove difficult for any administrator. Annette Grandin described the time, stating, "We went through some stormy days during her reign."

The root of the problem was that two distinct corporate cultures tried to blend together without ever making a commitment to be one school. On one hand, Brethorst pointed out that fifty-six percent of the Mounds-Midway faculty were former students and that "there are aunt and niece combinations in important positions." On the other hand, MMSN could note that its graduates ranked tenth in the state in 1952 (out of twenty-eight nursing programs) while Asbury was a mere twentieth. Student work assignments, she insisted, should be made by the faculty and not by the hospital. Finally, Brethorst stated that the schools needed to "bring about a greater unification of purpose" to overcome "those nurses in the service areas who are in some cases 'silent objectors.'"[13]

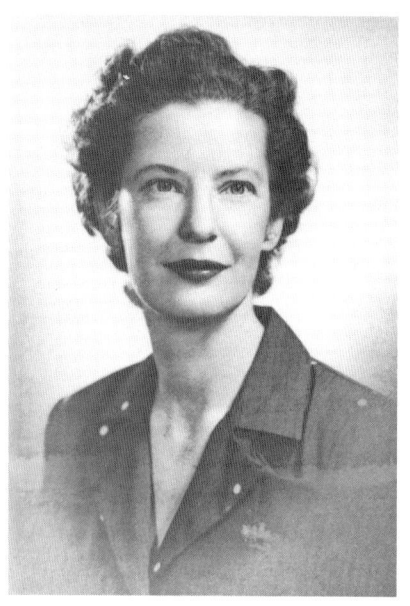

Daphne Rolfe

80 THIS CAP OF WHITE

Brethorst retired in 1952, replaced by Daphne A. Rolphe, who held the post until 1960. The new dean, a tall, elegant woman, was British, born in Cornwall, and receiving a nurse's diploma from the American Hospital in Paris, France. She furthered her education in the United States, earning a master's degree from Columbia University in New York in 1950. Although she remained somewhat distant to the students, maintaining offices at Hamline, she is remembered as gracious. Genevieve Sutton Brace recalled a special kindness. "Shortly before entering Hamline in the summer of 1952, I became engaged to Ray Brace, whom I met at Bethel. During my second year, we decided to marry the next summer if I could get permission. Dean Rolfe was supportive and arranged for me to transfer to the Asbury Division of Hamline for my senior year."

This, however, also shows the barriers that existed. Asbury and Mounds-Midway had separate traditions, separate choirs, separate yearbooks, and separate standards of conduct.[14]

The Education of a Nurse, 1950s

The Mounds-Midway Division, Hamline University School of Nursing, now had a single new class each year, beginning in June with science classes on the Hamline campus. This included residence at Manor House, a grand Tudor-style dormitory that lacked air-conditioning. Classes were held in "Old Main" and in the science building.

Many from those first classes remember the mixed feelings of anticipation and dread as they gathered at Hamline at the beginning of the summer. Most of them had just finished high school, but many had been working to save for fees for student uniforms and books. Some had attended institutions of higher learning — Bible schools or colleges. All suffered together through that long hot summer, certain that they would not be at the Midway dorm when fall arrived.

The summer course work proved challenging, as students were thrown into the difficult science courses. These included:

Course (Hours)	Class	Lab	Credits
Biology I, (anatomy and physiology)	36	72	4
Chemistry 10, (chemistry)	36	36	3
Biology III, (bacteriology)	36	36	3
Nursing (Ethics)	31	18	1
Total	126	144	11

"I had a big problem with chemistry," Valerie Buchan (1957) recalled. "I had to have tutoring and I asked the instructor, 'Am I ever going to need to know this?' He said, 'Don't you know what they're doing? They're separating the sheep from the goats.'" There were always a few casualties after the summer. Beginning in 1956, though, new students entered in September, then took "pre-nursing" classes during the fall semester at Hamline while living at the Midway nurses' dorm.

Nursing Arts

In the fall, following a one-week vacation, the new students then headed to Midway Hospital to begin clinical training. In that first year, students were placed in the care of Violet Nelson to learn how to become a nurse. She had a precise vision of what a nurse should be and her rules were drilled into young minds and often remained lodged there fifty years later. Everything mattered: how you made the bed, folded the towels, opened the blinds, arranged the flowers, brushed a patient's hair.

Violet Nelson drilled the fundamentals of nursing into those impressionable minds that, years later, they were not forgotten. Janet Valine Larson (1951) remembered, "We were taught perfection. If we cleaned it — it was perfect.

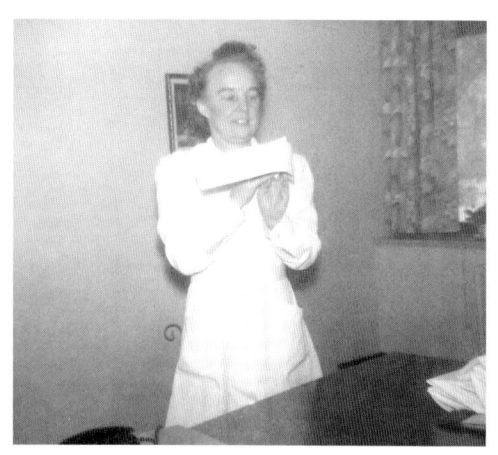

Violet Nelson shows the proper way to maintain a cap — sometimes referred to as "nellie bonnets."

There were no fitted sheets on hospital beds then. When we changed the linen, Miss Violet Nelson taught us the correct way to fold them, and how to hang them over a chair, while remaking a bed. Throwing linen on the floor was unheard of. The folds in the sheet hanging on a chair must face the hallway, so appearance from the hall was neat. No uneven edges showed." Joan Carlson Stolp (1951) added, "Don't you always have the closed end of the pillowcase facing the door of the room? I'm sure that you never . . . remove a jar lid and place it face down on a table."

Rachel Ostrom Lindahl (1957) described some of the principles: "Miss Nelson would peek in from behind the curtain when we were giving a bed bath and put her finger in the hot water to make sure it was the right temp. She taught us how to give a good back rub, we gave them twice a day in those years. I remember my first back rub was to a man who had so much hair on his back that I couldn't get the lotion off. It became a mass of matted hair."

Students were referred to as "Miss" rather than the familiar first name. This carried over to the patients, as Eula Marienau Stevenson

(1954) recalled. "In our nurses' lab, we were being taught how to give a bath. Our patients were fellow classmates. I referred to my patient by her first name, for which I was promptly reprimanded by Miss Nelson."

There were two attitudes towards Miss Nelson. Mary Jo Borglund Monson (1954) reminisced, "She was an example of perfection and expected and accepted nothing less than excellence from her students. And as she taught the arts of nursing, we learned and used those principles and procedures in our clinical experience and continue with those same arts in our daily lives."

Other students chafed under her stricture, wondering whether the larger picture was sometimes lost in the strict adherence to details. "There was only black and white with Miss Nelson," one former student stated. Lamenting the reliance on rote memorization, another graduate, who later took courses in a B.A. program, said, "We did not need to repeat all the procedures and all the steps of nursing care as often as we did."

Whatever view one had of Miss Nelson, there was no question that she instilled a sense of professionalism — that being a nurse was one of the most important of all vocations. And she lived that way. In later years, after she left Minnesota, she went back to school and earned the Master of Science in Nursing, then helped to develop an associate degree program at Modesto Junior College in California. In her sixties, she took a position at the American Baptist Hospital in Managua, Nicaragua and reorganized their school of nursing. After that, retired, she assisted with the development of a school of nursing at Bacone College — a Baptist school for Native Americans in Muskogee, Oklahoma.

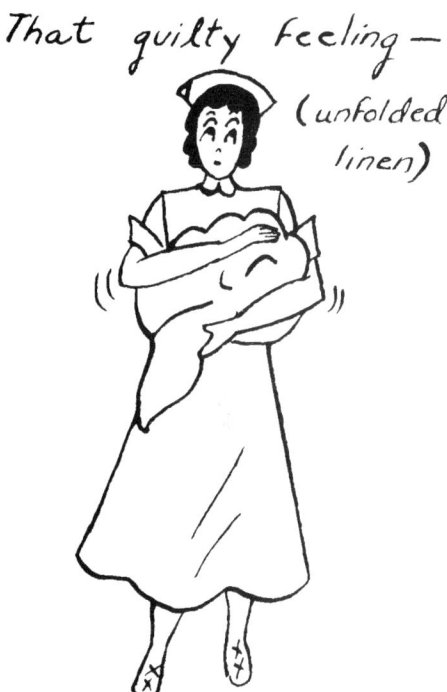

Capping

If the student survived the early months, with its hectic schedule and demanding coursework, they were ready to move beyond the "prelim" or "probie" stage. As Adella Bennett Espelien (1952) noted, with better admission standards, enhanced by standardized testing, the traditional vetting process of a probationary period lost much of its meaning. Although capping became more of a symbol rather than a mark of success, its emotional impact remained strong. Held in January or February, the ceremony was held at the Hamline Methodist Church during these years, typically attended by friends and family.

Barb Drier Kruschke (1954) described the feelings of the evening.

> At five o'clock, there's a feeling of excitement in the air, and everyone is watching for her folks and friends. There is a rush of crisp blues and whites in capless heads, as everyone is getting ready. The bus picks up forty-eight freshman from Midway and takes us to Hamline Methodist Church. There, our wonderful, big sisters meet us and settle the woozy feeling in our stomach by talking to us. The basement is a flutter of blue and white, as we are lined up and roses are pinned to our uniforms.
>
> As the processional begins, and our class marches down the aisle, it is then I feel that I have reached one of my goals as a nurse. The students take their seats and listen attentively. I shall never forget the impression Dr. Akenson made on me of my duties to man and God in my care of the sick. He said, "We have been called to do God's duty and to do it well. The nurse must first have a love for Christ, for the one without Him, cannot serve his patients well."
>
> The capping process started, and as my turn drew near, I thrilled at the thought of receiving my cap. As Miss Nelson placed the cap on my head, I thought of the new responsibility we were all taking on. With the light from our candles burning brightly, we all recited the Nightingale Pledge. We "promise to serve faithfully" in our profession in nursing. Following the capping, a reception was held, and after the congratulations, we introduced our friends and parents to teachers and supervisors.

Above: Harriet Peterson Danielson (1939) caps her daughter, Joanne Danielson Crocker (1964).

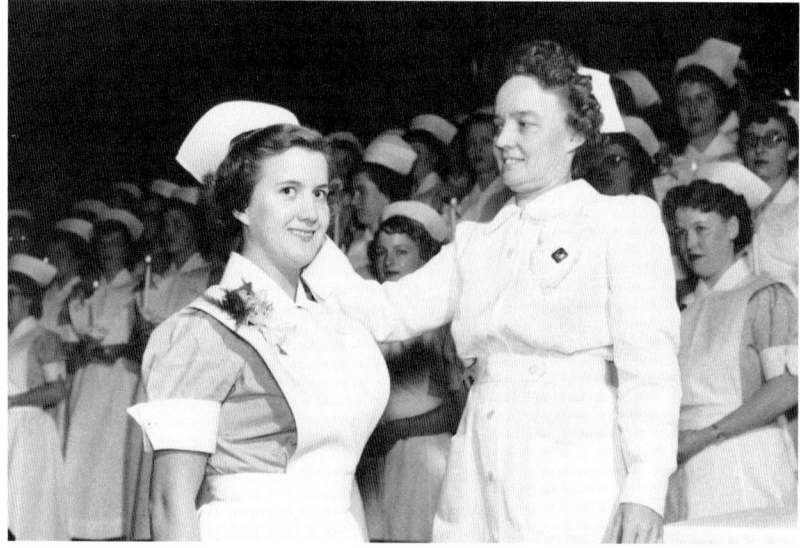

Right: Violet Nelson caps Marilyn Oliver Ames (1954)

Capping also had a more practical effect, because, now wearing the cap, the new student did not stand out as they walked the halls.

Classes and Clinicals

Students now fell into the pattern of a forty to forty-four hour week, replete with days and nights of work and study. The heart of the teaching method was the clinical rotations, in which an instructor was sometimes joined by a doctor or floor nurses.

OB proved memorable. Students had the opportunity to witness the miracle of birth then provide care for the newborns and mothers — who stayed in the hospital for as many as eight days in the 1950s. Carol Danielson Larson (1960) summarized the experiences as she looked back, writing, "I still remember my three months in OB at Midway. Each morning in the newborn nursery, the head nurse would lead us in prayer for each baby and mother in our care. Babies in distress were prayed for by name, mothers with pressures or problems were also named and we, as students were prayed for as we met new challenges and helped to form opinions about the quality of care at Midway. Now that I am older, I can more fully appreciate the power of prayer and I realize what a wonderful blessing that was for all involved."

One teacher often mentioned for the quality of her teaching was Thelma Hemmes, who came to Midway in 1949, and taught OB with a gentle manner that left the student understanding what needed to be done, but more importantly, why. Gena Testa Schottmuller (1957) remembered some of the lessons, "This is the mom's time to be treated

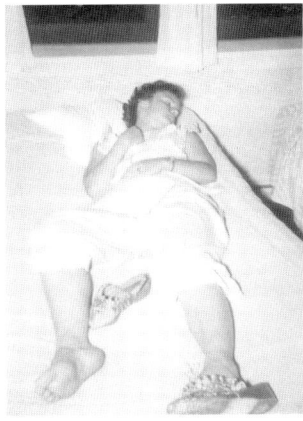

Virginia (Ginger) Gilbert (1952) studying for an exam.

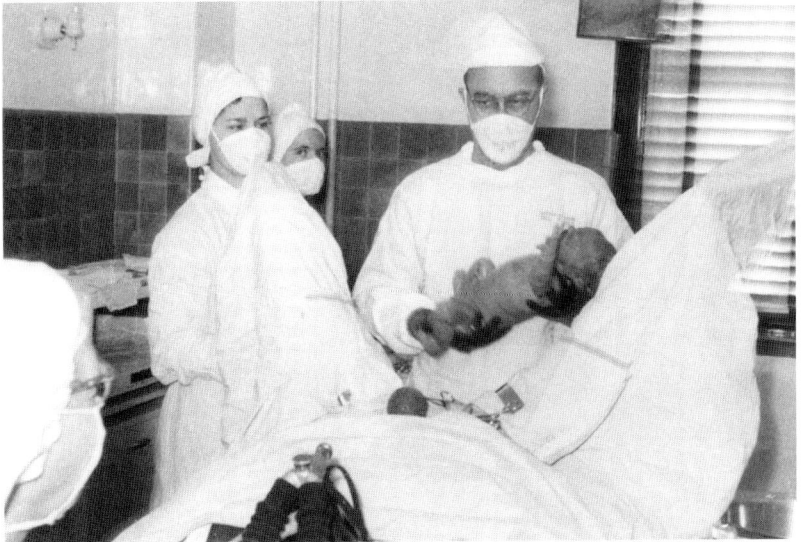

First delivery for student nurse Della Hildahl Fast (1954). Miss Lillo, R.N., is in the background and the physician is Dr. Walter.

like a queen. When she gets home, she will be working day and night so while she is here, there will be no time restrictions on the visitor unless the patient requests. When she goes home and has visitors she has to make them coffee and here we can do that for her. When her light goes on, be there to answer. Never walk by a patient's light."

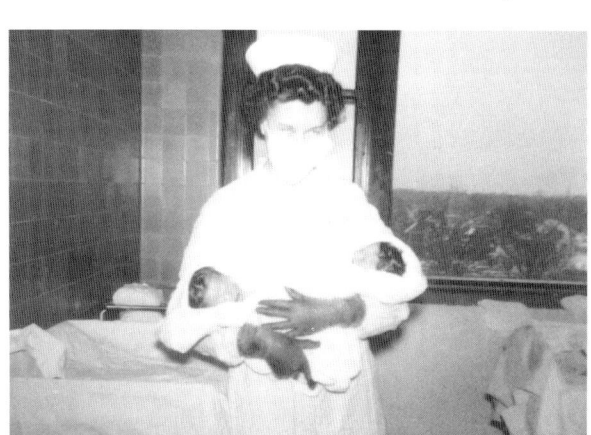

Thelma Hemmes holds twins.

Miss Hemmes also could be an advocate for the student, as Cordelia Kuhn Alfaro (1960) recalled, "I remember her backing me up one night after a physician threw a bedpan across the delivery room in a temper tantrum. To my knowledge, he never repeated that performance."

Genevieve Sutton Brace (1955) wrote about her "good fortune" to have Hemmes as maternity nursing instructor. Brace went on: "She recognized both weaknesses and strengths in her students. Although she needed to reprove me for my failure to adequately prepare for one clinical experience, in another instance she detected my strong interest in acquiring knowledge and developing skill. She not only assigned me to care for a patient with a rare postpartum disorder, she closely supervised and encouraged my efforts. I was enabled to implement "Therapeutic Use of Self", long before ever learning of that concept as a Nursing Intervention."

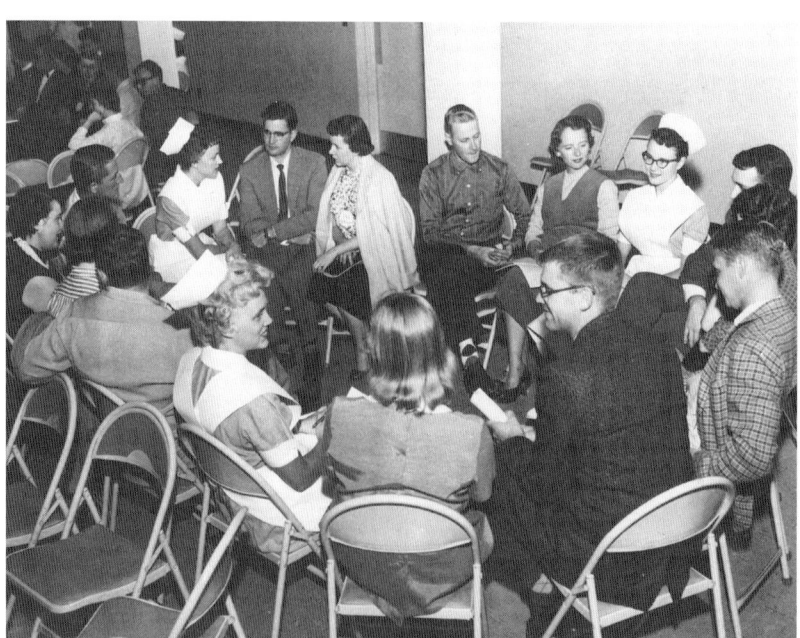

Parenting class, 1957

The impact was lasting, Alfaro said. "I continued on in Obstetrics and Gyn for twelve years after graduation and have Miss Hemmes to thank for knowledge, leadership, expectations, management of staff and a desire to keep learning." Brace echoed those sentiments, writing, "Miss Hemmes had a significant impact on my eventual decision to pursue a B.Sc. at the University of Minnesota, majoring in Nursing Education with a focus on Obstetrics. In subsequent years, I have come to highly value her role modeling, and appreciate her expertise."

If OB was "interesting, rewarding, mostly cheerful," as Alfaro remembered, it was also sometime "extremely sad." She gave an example: "I remember a multipara patient with extremely thin uterine wall. Neither parent would consider a hysterectomy or tubal ligation. The mother died one week after discharge and left several children motherless. A sobbing father returned to the unit with candy for us, wondering what he would do next, yet thanking us for what we had previously done."

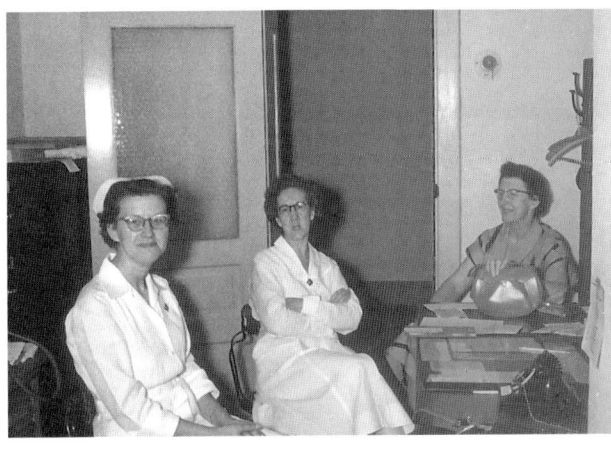

Lucille Kirsten, Esther Garnett, Edith Hammargren, July 1954

Of the many families that stepped through the doors, hoping for a glimpse of a newborn child, some of the most memorable visits were for Dr. Friedman's patients. He was Jewish but liked the care given at Midway. As one student recalled, "They would have a big room, and after eight days, the rabbi would come, joined by everyone's families, and perform a circumcision. And three or four of the family members would pass out."

A good instructor/student relationship was a two-way street, with the teacher sharing in the joy of learning. Barbara Carlson Dahl (1950) was clinical instructor in obstetrics at Midway Hospital. She reminisced, "I really enjoyed those years helping the students as they shared the happiness of new parents. My biggest reward from those years is to realize that I had the privilege of not only teaching nursing skills but of shaping lives. Many years after our time together on the third floor, a former student said to me, 'Thank you! Remember when I was ready to quit nursing? Your encouragement helped me to go on.'"[15]

Of all the rotations, none made a bigger impact than the three months in psychiatric nursing at Mounds Park. The hospital, of course, was renowned for its program and drew both short term and long-term patients, coming from many states like the Dakotas, Montana, Wyoming, and Wisconsin, as well as Canada.

Eleanore Anderson Vogel (1950), who joined the faculty in 1956, described the program:

> Emphasis was on assisting the patient to talk about their problems, what they planned to do about them and how to resolve feelings. These were brought about by encouraging good nutrition, activating patients with walks, occupational therapy and social parties, many one-to-one and one-to-group relationships, afternoon naps, back rubs, and body packs. Therapies included psycho-therapy, electro-shock therapy, insulin shock therapy, a few prefrontal lobotomies, sleep therapy, ultra-violet back massage, and sedative body packs.

Of course, to these young women, many still in their teens, the patients offered many memorable experiences. Jennie Larsen Just (1957) wrote: "I remember the compassionate care that was given and the small town neighborhood that existed at Mounds. A very strong memory . . . was the insulin shock therapy that was being done at that time and I can close my eyes and remember that fruity smell as the patients were being tubed in the early morning hours to bring them out of the insulin induced shock."

There were occasions that lingered in the student's thoughts. One member of the class of 1952 recalled their initiation into the psych wards: "There was one in the wards, a longtime patient, who, when the probies came, he got all of the men to get up on their hands and knees and bark like dogs. Scared us half to death." Lauralie Nelson Robertson (1950) remembered, "While working on first floor psych ward, a patient came out to me and said, 'I can see through you. My husband is an x-ray technician.'"

Many students refer to the awesome responsibility that was handed to them. One member of the class of 1952 said, "The summer between my freshman and junior year, I spent in charge of ground floor psych at Mounds at night. That was scary. I was putting two and three patients in insulin shock at five in the morning. By myself."

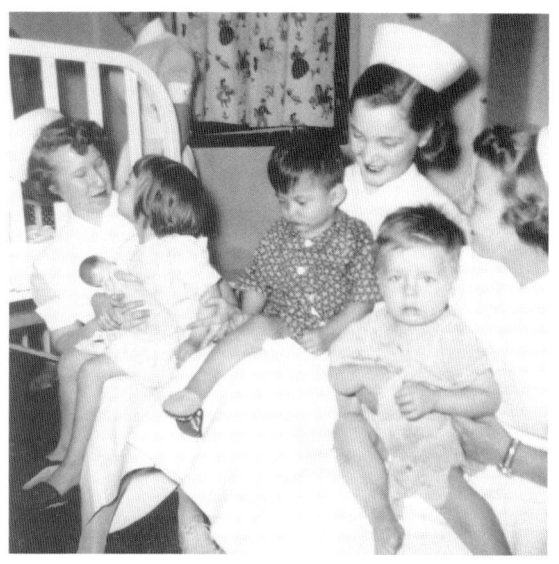

Pediatrics at Ancker Hospital. Margery Siemans, Char Erdmann, Beverly Biebighauser (1954)

Others remembered taking patients for walks through nearby parks or even taking them downtown Saint Paul. Jolyn Conrad Vigen (1954) remembered, "There was one long-term resident, an heiress, who did everything to push your buttons. She had a lot of privileges and could go to movies or go shopping. But she would always do something to embarrass you — pass gas, belch, or talk loudly in the middle of a quiet scene in a movie."

The contagion/communicable disease rotation was given at Ancker Hospital, where students mingled with those from other programs and lived in a dorm with less supervision than they were used to at Midway or Mounds. Patients included those who suffered from tuberculosis — often older men, who might sit out in the sun as part of the treatment, and occasionally shout out at the passing student nurses.

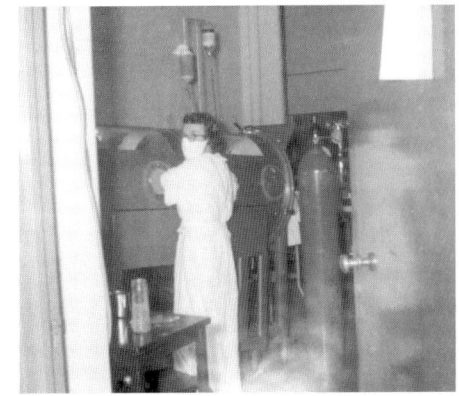

Gracia Riedell (1957) working with a polio patient in iron lung at Ancker Hospital.

The United States experienced an outbreak of 58,000 polio cases in 1952, followed by 35,000 cases in 1953, up from a typical number of around 20,000 cases a year. "If you came down with a fever, you were worried," one student said. During these years, the wards were filled at Ancker.

Some suffered from permanent respiratory paralysis and were placed in an iron lung. Mary Jo Borglund Monson (1954) recalled one young mother who had polio, and was in a respirator. "She could not take her eyes off the plug of the iron lung," Mary Jo said, "knowing that her life depended on it." Others remember working with patients, applying hot wool towels in the treatment method popularized by Sister Kenney. "I was so happy," Jolyn Conrad Vigen recalled, "when Salk came out with his vaccine."

Cordelia Kuhn Alfaro recalled,

> I am now working in Infection Control, many years after Birgit Tofte's lessons in contagion, but I still remember the basics. I experienced families being cured and reunited after TB treatment, children surviving measles, but dying of staph infections, polio and iron lungs and a small child admitted with mastoiditis, neglected as to care and symptoms prior to admission. The mother was an alcoholic and she stood by the crib, at night, drunk, and crying. The child lived, but was discharged home with her after an extensive hospital stay. I often wonder what happened to the child.

Other students gravitated toward surgery, enjoying the challenge of working with the doctors and highly-skilled nurses in often tense circumstances.

Ruth Huber Baxter (1954) said, "My favorite rotation was the surgery department with supervisor Agnes Sidlo. She made surgery so interesting and took the fear away from us, as we entered the department for work. I was in the first group to go through the surgical rotation and our first day on duty, three of my companions fainted. Miss Sidlo said she had no stretchers left to care for any more students who may faint during surgery."

Gena Testa Schottmuller (1957) fondly remembered surgery with Bernice Sjernstrom, writing:

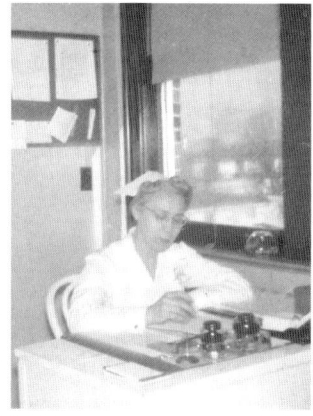

Agnes Sidlo

- Folding linens a special way so that every fold was perfect as each item was stacked. (This practice influences the way I fold my clothes today). These linens were then used in packs which we made up for every case.
- Stretching gauze. These were pieces of gauze which were previously used on another patient. They were washed, dried on boards with pins on all four sides, then folded in a special way so no loose ends were seen.
- The needles were used and reused after flushing with soap and water and alcohol. Some of them had burrs on them which then had to be removed. We would run each needle on a sharpener and smooth out the burr.
- Always being reminded of how important it was to do the work

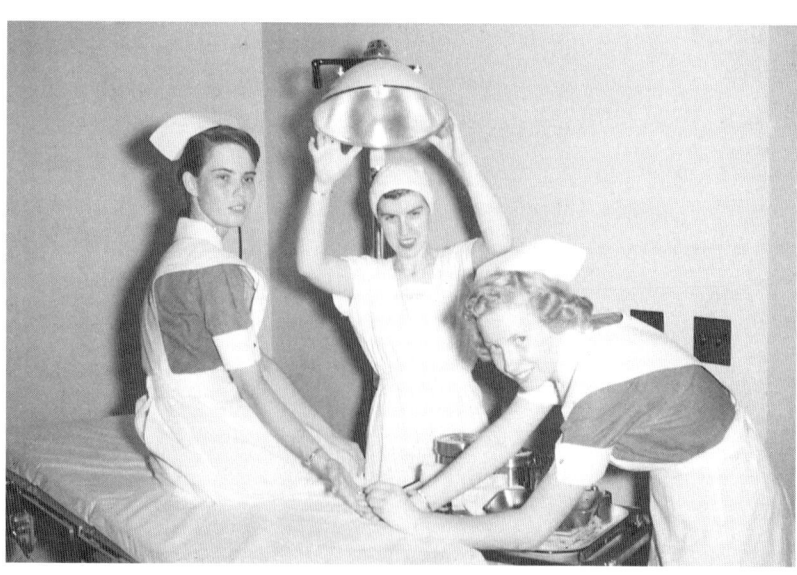

Fay Dalton, Vonna Shearer Ledeboer, Betty Wolfangle Breitenfeldt at Mounds Park Hospital, 1952

ready to be done and not wait until after lunch or another time.
- She would encourage us to 'never put off until tomorrow what you can do today.'

Sterilization was the unbreakable rule in surgery. Lillian Bloom May (1952) was acting as the instrument nurse for Dr. Grau and Dr. Williams at Midway Hospital during an appendectomy. When the doctors said they were ready, she turned to bring the instrument table over the patient and, not seeing the sponge pail, she accidentally fell over it onto the floor, but all the time keeping her sterile gloved hands in the air. The supervisor, Miss Sidlo, came into the surgery room and saw this student on the floor with her arms in the air and both doctors laughing with tears running down their faces. The student exclaimed, "But my hands are sterile!" At this, the supervisor exclaimed that "it would be best to change the gloves anyway."

Gracia Riedell (1957) remembered one night when she was called to assist with an appendectomy and found out that it was with Dr. John Earl. "I thought, this is like the right hand of God. But he was so nice, letting me scrub in and hold stuff and feel a part of it." She concluded, "Even God's come down and remember when they were students." He was, said another, the ideal of what a doctor should be.

Rural nursing, a new clinical experience, began in 1950, partly driven by a requirement that Minnesota state scholarship students spend six weeks in a rural hospital. Mounds-Midway

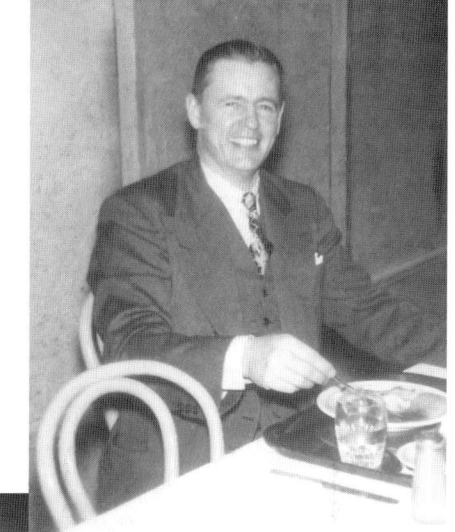

Above: Dr. John Earl

Left: Charlotte Sandin Olson demonstrates med/surg technique. In 1971, Olson returned to Mounds-Midway as its last director.

Chapter Three 91

students worked in hospitals in Benson, Bemidji, Crookston, Hibbing, Grand Rapids, Stillwater, St. Cloud, Thief River Falls, and Worthington. Students learned about the various social and health organizations while they were in the hospital and after they were discharged. They learned about the people in the community, their way of life, and their social and economic background.

There are many fond memories of this rotation. Valerie Buchan (1957) said, "Three of us went to Thief River Falls. We worked at the hospital and the little town welcomed us. We were constantly asked out for dinner." This happened in every small town visited by the student nurses, leading Arvis Eastland to write, "Most of the girls found rural nursing to be quite a social whirl." She further noted, "Of course, not everyone was in as big a demand as Borgie." Indeed, Mary Jo Borglund, who went to Stillwater in December 1953 for her rotation, had a particularly rewarding time in rural nursing. One fellow, David Monson, was suffering from mononucleosis, but as his health improved, they found a mutual attraction. They were engaged on June 6, 1954, the day Mary Jo graduated from Mounds-Midway School of Nursing, and married that October.[16]

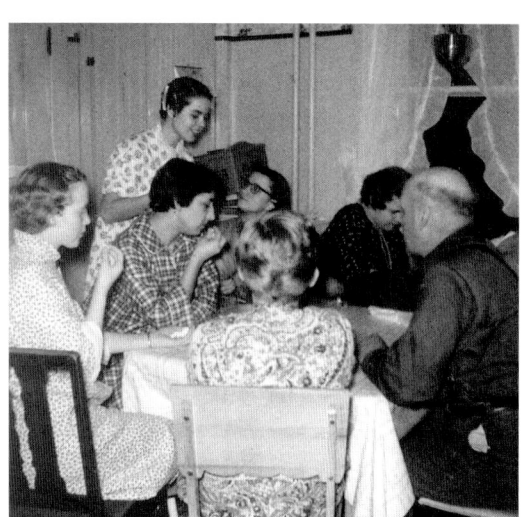

Rural nursing in Bemidji, February 1957. Gena Testa Schottmuller, seated in the middle, and Iona Stone Holsten, standing (both 1957).

The Life of a Student Nurse, 1950s

Mary Jo Borglund Monson (1954) described it best, when she said, "We lived together. We bonded like sisters. We faced life and death together." Valerie Buchan called it "a strange sort of sisterhood."

One thing that students got used to were the long hours with split shifts, at first a forty-four hour, then forty hour week. The two campuses required many trips on the bus or streetcar. "We went to classes at both Mounds Park and Midway Hospital, usually taking the streetcar back and forth. If we happen to be working nights, we still attended our day classes, where ever they were scheduled," Janet Valine Larson (1951) said.

Myrtle Anderson Hoffpauir (1955) added,

> One of my many memories being a student at Mounds-Midway was the traveling between hospitals on our rotations. We had to go by streetcar most of the time. Carrying all those suitcases and other things made for a big challenge. Since I did a lot of sewing,

92 THIS CAP OF WHITE

my parents gave me a portable sewing machine for my high school graduation. Lugging that machine around was something I will never forget! I think it weighed forty pounds! I don't remember how many trips I had to make to get all my things to the next hospital, but I know it was too many.

There were now new dorms at Mounds and Midway, following the opening of the new building on Aldine in 1951, so that housing became slightly more comfortable. Still, rules were kept. While faculty had previously served as housemothers, mature women were hired to watch over the young students at Midway. At Mounds, though, faculty still kept their vigils.

Lauralie Nelson Robertson (1950) wrote, "While at Midway, lights were to be out at ten p.m. and Annette Grandin came and checked up on us with her flashlight. Many a night, I put my hair up in the dark." If you happened to be out, the ten p.m. deadline could loom over the evening festivities. Rachel Ostrom Lindahl (1957), recalled, "The door was locked at that time and if we came in late, the house mother had to be awakened. None of us wanted that." There were alternatives, as one member of the class of 1952 said: "I had a ground level room and we had a regular traffic jam some nights."

With all the hard hours of work and study, often in a cloister-like atmosphere, it is not surprising that occasionally, students found ways to add some spark to their life. Ruth Huber Baxter (1954) wrote, "We had curfew hours and often we got caught trying to stretch those hours. One of my housemothers was Mrs. Malmberg. Many pranks were pulled on her, and especially the one when she found a skeleton under her bed. There are still detectives working on that case."

Marilyn Moberg Benson (1957) wrote, "I had a family antique to school with me. My big Ben alarm clock, which rang extra loud, and belonged to my dad. I had a hard time keeping track of it. One evening, it found its way into our house mother's apartment and hid under her bed to ring at three a.m." To Marilyn's surprise, when she asked about her "missing" clock in the office the next day, it was returned without questions.

She also remembered sneaking the demonstration dummy, named Annie, out of the basement class laboratory. She wrote, "We sat her by the telephone in the hallway of our dorm so our housemother would see her when she made rounds to make sure we were all in our rooms at the ten o'clock curfew. When ten o'clock came, there was the house

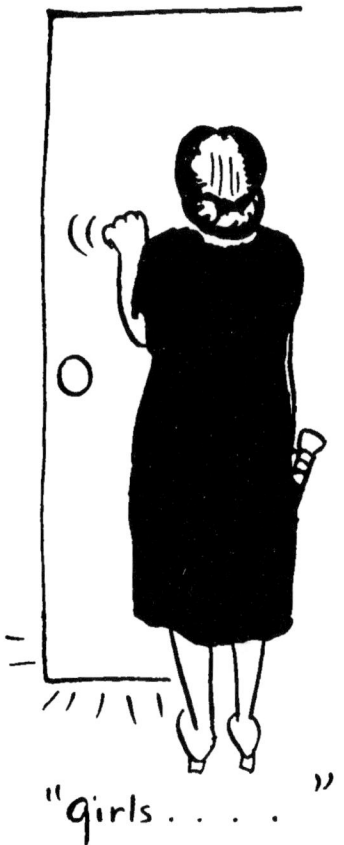

"girls...."

Chapter Three 93

Grape Pudding
Affectionately known as
"Grape Glop"
served in the Mounds Park
Dining Room

Ingredients:
2 cups blue grape juice
2 T. cornstarch
3 T. sugar
3 T. water
¼ t. salt
Combine sugar, cornstarch, salt, and water in saucepan. Heat grape juice and slowly stir into other ingredients. Cook and stir over low heat until mixture is clear and thick. Serve cold with dollop of whipped cream.

mother scolding the dummy for not being in her room—thinking it was a real person! It was so funny listening to her talk to Annie. We girls had our heads buried in our pillows to keep our laughter muffled until the housemother left."

Cordelia Kuhn Alfaro (1960) recalled similar pranks with her roommate, Beverly Wall Jessup (1960).

> One time, at Mounds Hospital, we removed all of the furniture from her room as a prank, because we knew she was getting "pinned" that night. I don't think she spoke to us for a week! We played the trumpet on different floors, rolled pumpkins and watermelons down the halls and played pranks on the housemother at Midway. Somehow she continued on as housemother in spite of our antics. One night we cut one of the girl's long black hair and promptly pasted it on Mrs. Chase, the demo mannequin. Miss Nelson was not "happy" the next morning when she had to teach a freshman class basic techniques, using that mannequin.

Food always brought variety to life. Almost always. Joan Carlson Stolp (1951) recalled, "That wonderful weekly dessert we were supposed to believe was 'raspberry lemange'—we called it 'grape glop.'" Others remember trips to Perry's on the corner near Mounds Park.

Community social life included seasonal parties, such as Halloween and Christmas. Special entertainment might include a class play, such as a production of Gilbert and Sullivan's *Mikado* or Dickens's *A*

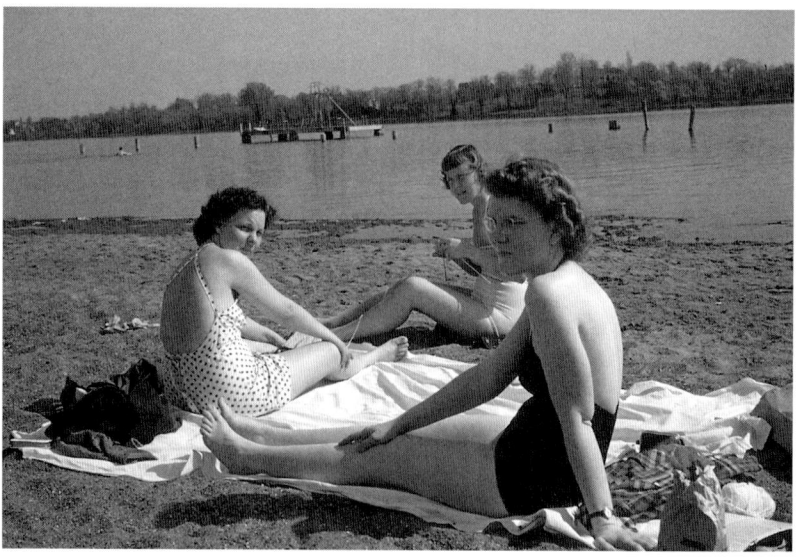

Ruth Biery, Ruby Eliason, and Alice Turk at the beach at Lake Phalen, May 1, 1952

Christmas Carol. Rachel Ostrum Lindahl (1957) recalled, "In our freshman year we put on a play called Snow White and the Seven Pituitary Deficiencies. I was Snow White because I was the tallest in our class, so that all the shorter girls could be the Pituitary Deficiencies."

Living in the city of Saint Paul, students found many pleasures in the surrounding neighborhoods. Jennie Larsen Just (1957) wrote, "Another reason that I really liked being at Mounds was the social life. We had wiener roasts at Phalen and swam at Tanner's Lake and it was there that I met my husband who grew up on McLean Avenue off of Earl Street. We walked all over the East Side of Saint Paul."

There were, of course, men in the lives of many students, although marriage was forbidden for students. A few exceptions were allowed by the late 1950s. In other instances, secret marriages were carried on for months, with the brides returning to the dorm to complete their three years.

Choir remained a source of enjoyment. Professor Jaeger continued to lead the group until 1954, when he retired, but not until he had conducted the choir on television for the first time in March 1952. His replacement, Bob Mantzke, opened up the repertoire from Jaeger's more traditional approach. Jo Ann Lewis Moberg (1958) wrote, "Bob Mantzke's direction brought us through a variety of musical styles. We sang at various area churches and were live on TV at Christmas time.

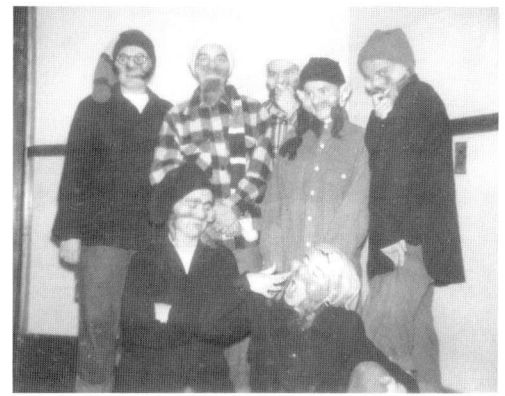

Snow White and the Seven Pituitary Deficiencies. Mary Dobbertin (Doc), Marge Berg (Happy), Evelyn Severe (Sneezy), Gerry Austin (Dopey), Marilyn Larson (Bashful), Elsie Abrahamson (Grumpy), Jan Harris (Sleepy).

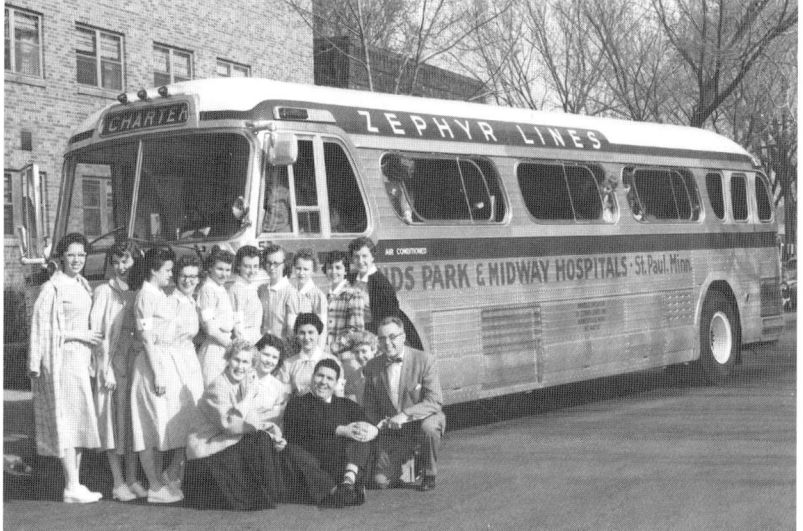

The choir goes on tour, 1957. Chaperones included Eleanore Anderson Vogel (1950), Bob Mantzke, director, and Dr. Horace Wood, director of public relations, Baptist Hopital Fund.

Chapter Three 95

Our spring trips were especially fun though not very long — only four days. They couldn't spare us from the hospital work force."

Singing was not just for choir members, though, as Janet Valine Larson (1951) recalled. "A fringe benefit for patients at both Mounds Park and Midway Hospital, was the students going on a.m. duty early Sunday mornings, singing hymns in the hallways. Some patients referred to us as angels, and there were those who thought it was much too early in the morning!"

Spiritual life

At the heart of the school was its commitment to Christian service. The school handbook, *The Lamplighter*, said the following:

> Attendance at morning chapel is an expected and required activity. Sunday morning singing in the hospital corridors is an inspiration to you and to our patients. The spirit of Christian service has always been closely linked with the practice of nursing. Your New Testament, which you will receive at capping, is to become a part of your uniform.

It was more than just rules, though, as students found a wonderful joy in the ability to share their spiritual journeys. Phyllis Bordwell Larson (1950) wrote, "I grew up in a rural community, and in a very small rural church, where our youth fellowship consisted of two or three, so fellowship with many Christian young women was truly a blessing."

Students could also turn to their instructors, as Gena Testa Schottmuller remembered,

> My spiritual growth was strengthened in the presence of other instructors and student nurses with whom I could pray, discuss concerns, and have them point out special scripture for my concerns. I'm thinking of a situation in psych rotation where I had much difficulty with a particular mentally ill patient. Eleanor Anderson, (now Vogel), instructor, was key in helping me work out my anxiety and pointed out scripture to assist me as well. "Peace I leave with you," John 14:27, was one of my favorites.

The spiritual life was encouraged through a variety of events and

In the Dorm

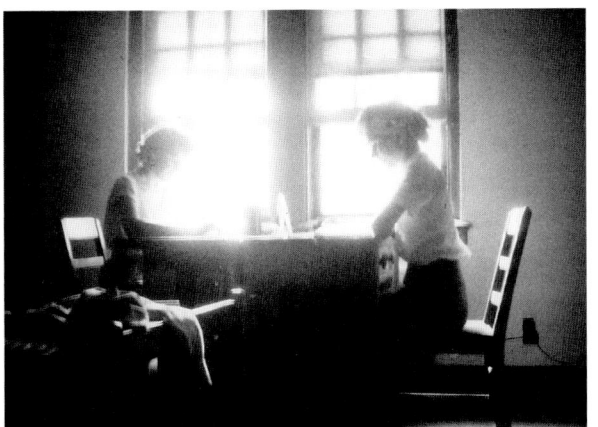

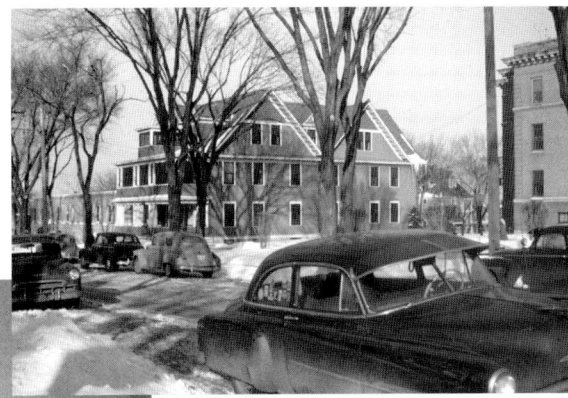

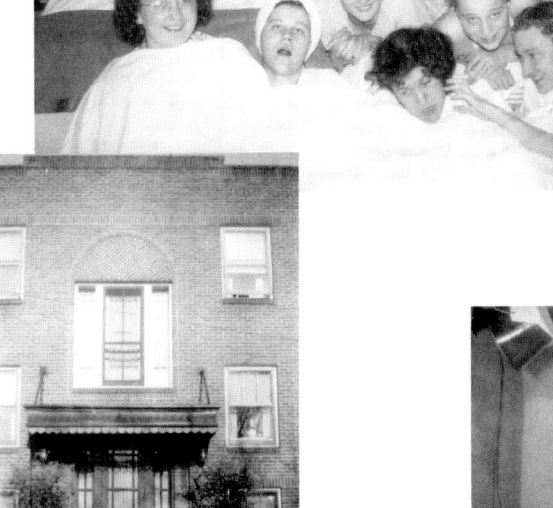

Above, left: Studying in the dorm at Hamline University. Above, right: Dorms at Mounds Park, 1952. Left: A gathering in Marge Berg and Adella Bennett Espelien's room

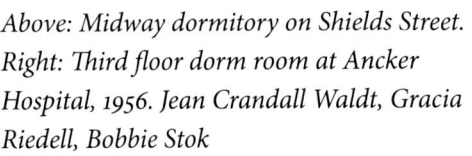

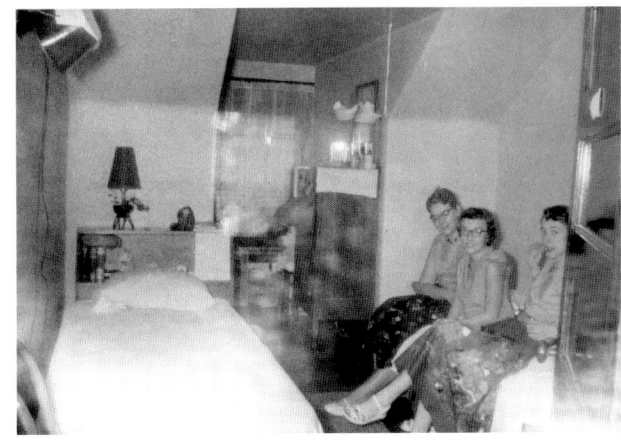

Above: Midway dormitory on Shields Street. Right: Third floor dorm room at Ancker Hospital, 1956. Jean Crandall Waldt, Gracia Riedell, Bobbie Stok

Chapter Three 97

The farewell tea was a tradition. Here, Muriel Severson, Ruth Gustafson, Violet Nelson, Lucille Kirsten, and Arlene Lick say goodbye to Elaine Westlund Coleman (1950).

meetings, including a widely-attended Nurses' Christian Fellowship and an annual Deeper Life Conference.

Janice Jackson Johnson (1953) summed up the feelings of many graduates when she wrote, "Recently I was looking through some of my old journals and other items. One of the items was a small black notebook I used during my time as a nursing student. Among other things, I rediscovered letters of encouragement from other students, poems, and notes from NCF meetings and retreats. During this time, I also found role models for living as I watched the lives of my fellow students and faculty."

Graduation

The classes through 1953 continued their graduation ceremonies as Mounds-Midway graduates. Traditions leading up to final days included keeping a chain of safety pins, then taking one off each day as the end grew closer. Others recall "ripping" when your dress was torn up after the last day on the floor as a student.

When the school became a division of Hamline, graduates participated in that school's ceremonies and the instructors marched with the University's faculty. Graduates received a diploma from Hamline University and were given a pin that combined the symbols of the white cross from Hamline-Asbury with the four-sided shape of the traditional Mounds-Midway pin. Many fondly recall that the nurses

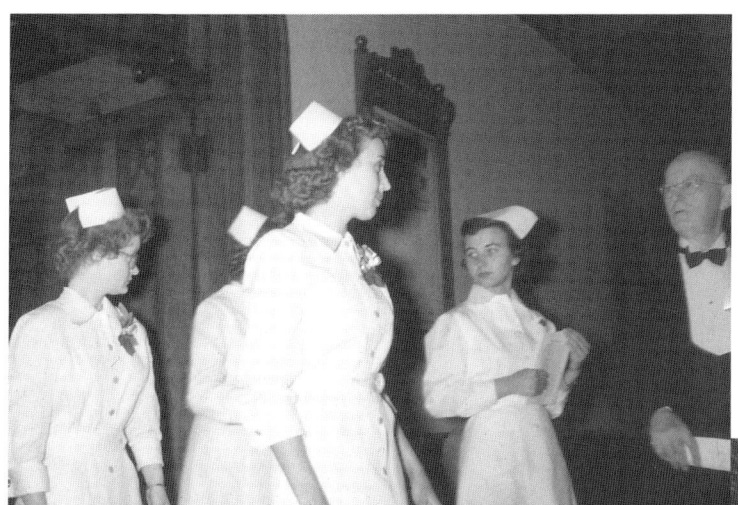

Graduation, 1950s

Left: Graduation, 1952, was held at the First Baptist Church, Saint Paul. This was the so-called "experimental class" that graduated before a complete merger with Hamline University.

Right: Graduation, 1960. This was the last class to graduate as part of Hamline University.

Below: Burning the blues at the last class picnic, 1954.

Chapter Three 99

did not don the traditional black gown, but marched into the field house first, proudly wearing their whites. Jolyn Conrad Vigen said, "People commented that the nurses stole the show."

These were special moments. Gracia Riedell remembered that although her father had not been supportive of her entry into nursing school, he took off work to attend her graduation. "And he never took off work," she said. "I was so proud that day."

The true end — the achievement of the long-sought goal — really came several months later. In August, graduates took the state boards, usually over two days, to qualify for the coveted title of Registered Nurse. As one student said, "The fear of God was put into us to pass the boards. It wasn't so much that you failed personally, but that you failed the whole school." Another 1957 graduate recalled, "I worked at St. John's and some students had taken the tests already. They told us that if you received a long envelope, you failed, and if you passed, the letter came in a small envelope. We went home looking for the mail every day and then I got a long envelope. I was afraid to open the letter, but I passed and later learned that everyone received the long envelope."

The Break

The union of Hamline University and the Mounds-Midway School of Nursing unraveled in 1957 following an accreditation visit from members of the National League for Nursing. Their report stated that finances, nursing faculty, and student personnel policies differed significantly from Hamline University policies. The choice had to be made, they insisted, or accreditation might be threatened. The NLN staff secretary questioned whether "any program not leading to a degree should be in a senior college."[17]

The impeding break was signaled in November 1957 when Mel Conley, longtime hospital administrator, informed the Minnesota Board of Nursing in a private letter of the intention to re-open the independent Mounds-Midway School of Nursing in the fall of 1958. The major impetus came from Hamline University following an internal evaluation that recommended that the college concentrate its resources and staff on the liberal arts program. This also meant the demise of the Asbury Hospital division. Since the hospitals heavily subsidized the Hamline program, the loss of income led to a decision to terminate the four-year degree nursing program at that school as well.

Mutually, the two schools agreed to go their separate ways, although, with students already in the program, the Hamline connection did not officially end until 1960 when they graduated.

The Baptist Hospital Fund (BHF) embraced the change. Both fundraising and school applications had dropped after Mounds-Midway lost its special bond to regional Baptist churches. In addition, a state board representative noted after a meeting with Mr. Conley, "Religion courses will probably be included in the curriculum. This has been one area in which there has been some dissatisfaction because of the difference in religion between the University and the clinic areas."

Back under the management of the BHF by the fall of 1958, the school was legally a new program and needed accreditation from the Minnesota Board of Nursing—which it received almost at once. Although other diploma schools began closing during these years, there seems to have been little debate that the school needed to continue. Indeed, the board clearly stated that "the field of nursing is a strategic opportunity for service to society on the part of Christian young women." Calling on the "ideals of devotion and service," its new mission statement included a call to "encourage qualified Baptist young women to enter the profession" and a commitment to assist "in the preparation of competent and dedicated nurses for missionary service throughout the world."[18]

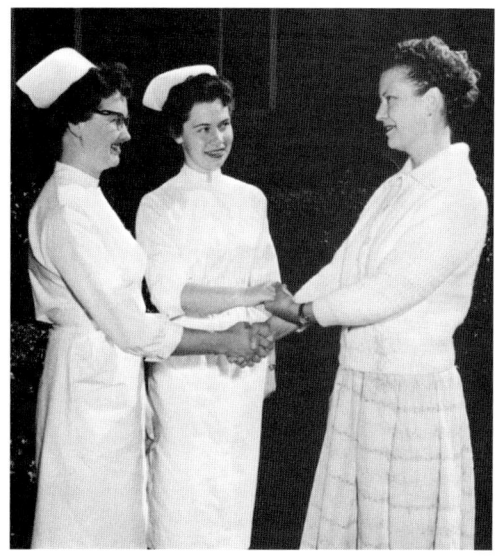

Joanne Wright, Karen Carlson, and Daphne Rolfe at 1960 graduation, Hamline University

One suspects that Mary Danielson would have been pleased with those goals. Following retirement in 1952, she continued to live at the dormitory at Mounds Park—except for an extended stay in the hospital following a heart attack. Upon her death in 1954, a newspaper reporter wrote:

> Mary Danielson is no longer here on earth as you and I are; the Lord took her home last July 14 after a long and busy and distinguished career in the dual role of hospital administrator and director of Mounds-Midway School of Nursing in St. Paul, Minnesota.
>
> Yet in a real way she still is here. They could not see her, it is true, but she was at Tezpur, India, on October 19 for the capping ceremony of the first six student nurses. Mounds-Midway graduate Arlene Jensen (Callaway, 1943), herself now the director of the Baptist Christian School of Nursing of Tezpur, Assam, told

Chapter Three 101

us so. Here are her words: "How thrilled they were to receive the caps. . . . We gave them Mounds-Midway caps and so we might say that the influence of Mounds-Midway School of Nursing and of Miss Danielson who led it so well for so many years, is still reaching the far corners of the earth."

There were other changes. Violet Nelson, after more than twenty years of teaching Nursing Arts, also left, heading to California to care for her mother. Ruth Gustafson stepped down as Mounds Park Hospital educational coordinator in 1955, although she continued to help with the school library.

So while the renewal of the Mounds-Midway School of Nursing seemed to be a return to older traditions, it was also the time for a new generation to step into key positions when many hospitals began to discontinue schools as uneconomical and many educators turned their backs on diploma schools. If Mounds-Midway was to survive into the 1960s and 1970s, it would require leadership and dedication.

Endnotes

[1] *Mounds-Midway School of Nursing Annual Report*, 1949.

[2] Esther Lucille Brown, *Nursing for the Future* (New York: Russell Sage Foundation, 1948), 45, 165.

[3] "Graham Davis attacks Brown Report on Nursing for the Future," *Modern Hospital*, 71 (October 1948), 138. Kenneth A. Brent, "Are Nurses Getting Too Much Education?" *Hospital Management*, 67 (April 1949), 68.

[4] "Survival of Hospital School Called Matter of Utmost Urgency," *Hospital Management*, 69 (January 1950): 30.

[5] Mary Danielson, 31 October 1936, in Espelien, p. 29.

[6] Correspondence, H. Schwartz, 15 December 1948, 23 February 1949.

[7] Correspondence, H. Schwartz, 15 December 1948, 23 February 1949.

[8] L. Christensen report, 3 June 1952.

[9] *Saint Paul Pioneer Press*, 31 May 1949; *Bulletin, Hamline University School of Nursing, 1950-1952*, 144.

[10] *The Watchman Examiner*, 4 September 1958.

[11] *Mounds-Midway School of Nursing Annual Report*, 1951.

[12] *Mounds-Midway News Letter*, 12 (November 1950), 4.

[13] *Report of the Dean of the Hamline University School of Nursing*, 6 October 1954. Hamline University Archives.

[14] *Minutes of the Coordinating Committee of the Hamline University School of*

[15] *Nursing*, 4 November 1953. Hamline University Archives.

[15] *Mounds-Midway School of Nursing Alumni Newsletter* (February 1996), 2.

[16] For a look at one community's view of the Rural Nursing course, see *Stillwater Gazette*, 9 June 2000.

[17] *Comments and Recommendations from the National League for Nursing Collegiate Board of Review*, 4 June 1957. Hamline University Archives.

[18] Wanyce C. Sandve to Leonora J. Collatz, executive secretary, Minnesota State Board of Nursing, 19 June 1958. Minnesota Board of Nursing, Minnesota Historical Society; *Mounds-Midway News Letter*, 18 (May 1958), 1.

CHAPTER FOUR
My Heart, My Mind

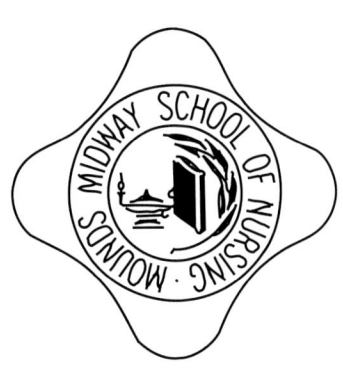

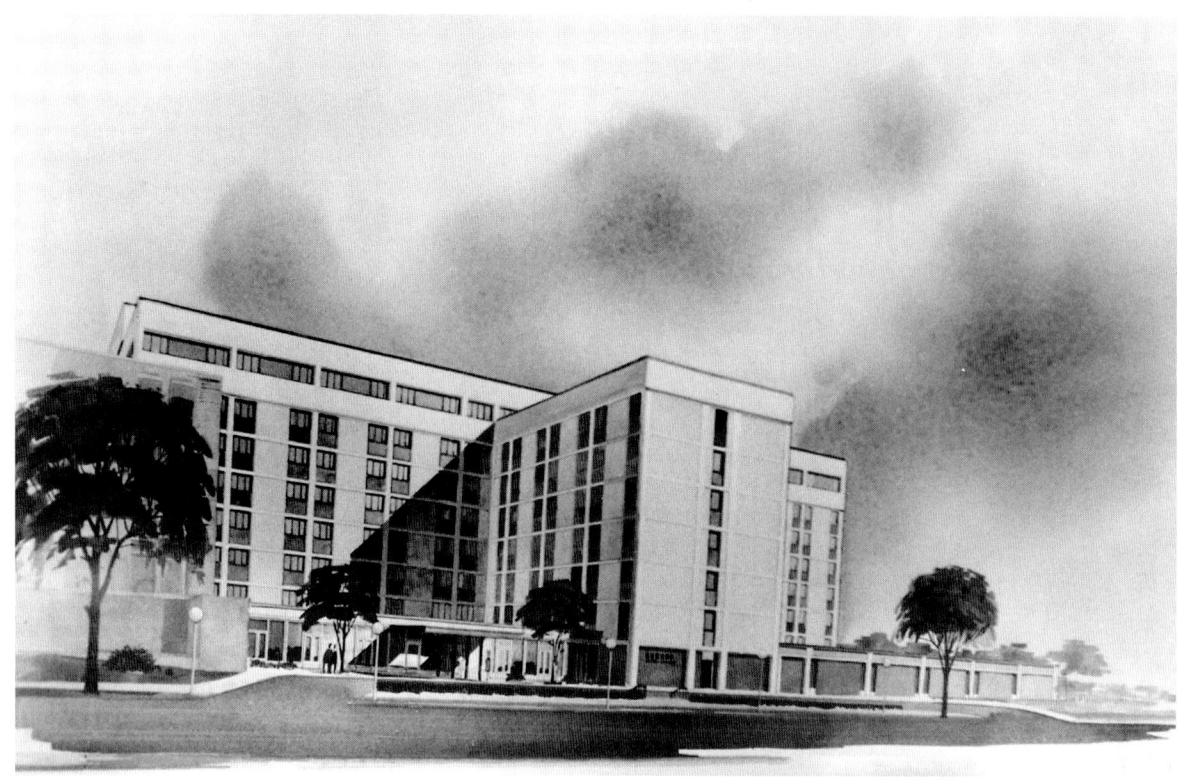

The "New" Midway

*I*N THE SUMMER OF 1958, Judith Anderson became the first student to enroll in the "new" Mounds-Midway School of Nursing. The hospital newsletter proudly declared, "Mrs. Wanyce Sandve, acting Director of the School of Nursing, has reported that inquiries have been received from coast to coast." The Baptist Hospital Fund (BHF), now solely in charge of the school, had turned to Sandve for leadership. She was a graduate of the University of Minnesota, and held a master's degree in public health. She had served as staff nurse in the psychiatric division at the University of Minnesota. For three years, she served as public health nurse of Isanti County, then for eleven years was on the faculty of the school of public health at the University of Minnesota. At the time of her appointment, she was instructor at Hamline.[1]

She was a somewhat unusual choice, since she was not a MMSN graduate, was a Seventh-Day Adventist at a Baptist school, and had a strong background in public health — a field typically not offered by diploma schools with their hospital orientation. That the BHF hired her suggests the deep respect that Dr. George Earl and the Baptist Hospital Fund held for her. As a professional, Adella Bennett Espelien 1952) recalled, "She brought the concept of listening to the program and that had never been taught." A co-worker from another organization, describing her leadership, said, "She just had a knack for drawing people together, and when you get good people together, you get good results." As a person, Arlys Deckert Schwabauer (1964), remembered Sandve as "intelligent, firm, yet very kind. She knew the students well. She would have the seniors over to her house for a party prior to graduation and everyone looked forward to that time. There was a special twinkle to her smile."[2]

As Mounds-Midway embarked on its return to independent status, the other key leader was Melvin Conley, executive director of the Baptist Hospital Fund. He attracted strong financial support from the American Baptist Convention and drew in influential board members, such as Norman Mears. Estelle Johnson recalled those years, saying, "How grateful I am for the wonderful working environment that Mr. Conley created and maintained for all who worked here."[3]

The Baptist Hospital Fund, influenced strongly by Conley and Dr. George Earl, threw its wholehearted support behind the nursing school. In 1959, Sandve told Carl Lundquist, president of Bethel College and Seminary, that the BHF board saw the school as important to public

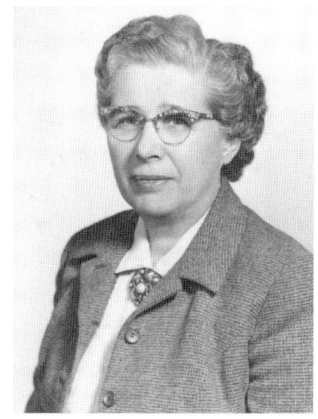

Wanyce Sandve

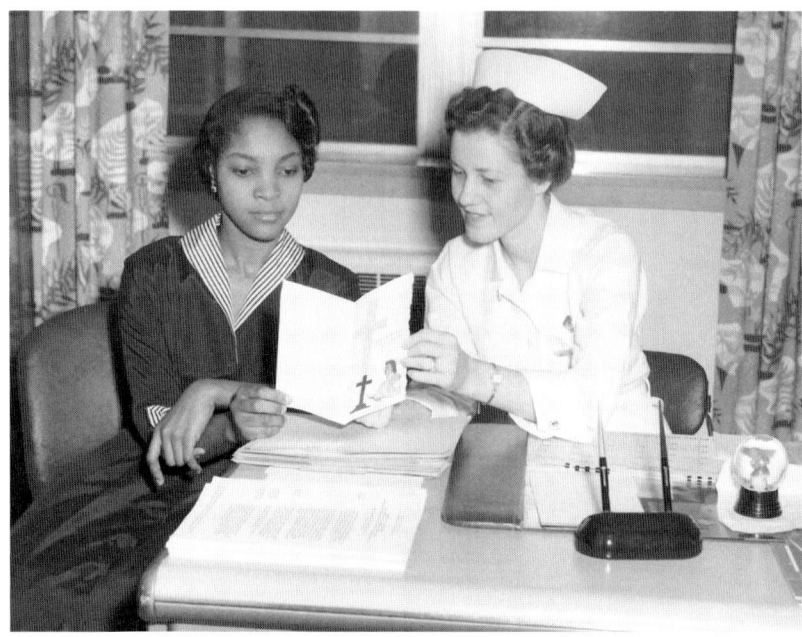

Magda Cadet Dumeny (1961) with Lillian Bloom May (1952). Magda, a native of Haiti, was a member of the first class admitted to the "new" Mounds-Midway.

relations benefit as they embarked on a major fundraising campaign for the two hospitals. Indeed, when the board endorsed its new long range plan in 1960, it included a major educational center. With the center, the Trustees stated, "School enrollment can be increased substantially and students will be afforded the opportunity for specialized clinical experience in the care of aging, health education, and in the use of the latest developments in constant care and rehabilitation." The plan anticipated a program for clinical training of ministers. While this grand plan led to substantial hospital construction at Mounds and Midway Hospitals, the dream of an expanded school of nursing quietly faded away.[4]

The Education of a Nurse, 1960s

The nature of nursing education was evolving, shaped by the tough professional standards of the National League of Nursing and the economic realities of hospital management. The direct link between training and work requirements was slowly being broken. In 1958, students had a forty-hour week, including classes, around sixteen hours of clinical practice (for "educational growth") plus twelve hours of nursing service for cost of board and room. Within a few years, students began to be paid for their work on the floors. The per-student expense to the school increased dramatically. This was made up by boosts to tuition charges, which were eased, in turn, by the increased availability of student loans. In one other significant change, married students were accepted by 1965.

Now independent from Hamline University, the Mounds-Midway faculty quickly formulated a new curriculum. Although based on the courses developed while a part of Hamline, it headed into several significant new directions. In an initial report, reviewers from the state nursing board offered praise for the curriculum committee:

> All three of these faculty members appear enthusiastic about their programs. One received the impression that they enjoyed working together and appear to share the planning and teaching. Mrs. Espelien takes responsibility for the majority of classroom teaching with Mrs. Erickson assisting her in demonstrations and supervision of practice in the laboratory. Miss Conrad spends most of her time in clinical areas with students. A wide variety of teaching methods are used and there seems to be much emphasis on student participation through such techniques as role-playing, individual or group investigation, and presentation.[5]

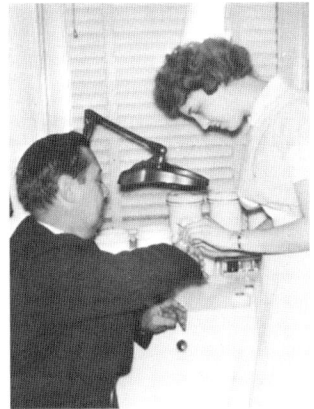

Industrial nursing, 1963

Sandve brought her expertise in public health to the curriculum, introducing new programs in public health and industrial nursing. She argued that "students need this experience extending into the community and gaining of knowledge of community health problems." Furthermore, she believed that with the rapid growth of the urban and suburban population after World War II, "the trend is toward urban nursing so the basic preparation of students of nursing should include health agencies in urban areas."

The school began a clinical rotation in Industrial Nursing in 1961, sending students to the Ford plant and the Whirlpool Corporation factory in Saint Paul. Taught by Fern Worm at Whirlpool and Ruth Miller at the Ford Plant, they reported, "Teaching the importance of nursing care in minor illnesses and injuries in order to keep the worker on the job was a new concept to the student."

Bonnie Erichsen Scherer (1962) recalled her time at the Ford plant,

> It was a great experience! If the wrong part came down the assembly line it was attached as the line didn't stop for anything. Then all the horns would honk all over the plant so everyone would know there was a mistake made. The only other time the horns would honk was when a student nurse walked by! We took a lot of steel

Chapter Four 109

splinters out of eyes and fingers, filed a lot of accident reports and insurance forms and passed out a lot of aspirins. I also learned how to catch a city bus at 5:30 am, transfer downtown St. Paul by myself and get to and from the Ford plant. I don't know how this 'fraidy cat survived being a student nurse!

The other new rotation was in outpatient clinical nursing. It began at Ancker Hospital, but was shifted in 1960 to the Wilder Dispensary in St. Paul—renamed the St. Paul Outpatient Center the following year. Here, under the guidance of Mrs. Kaufert, students learned about providing a broad range of community resources, including the opportunity to teach health classes. By the late 1960s, the clinical was taken "in-house" at Mounds and Midway. Some students also ventured into Emergency Room services. Cheryl McBride Dietrich (1970) recalled traveling by bus to Hennepin Emergency room in Minneapolis. She said, "We were able to put stitches in the drunks faces, under the direction of the ER doctor. We got to see a fast paced ER."

Still lacking a solid science curriculum since the Hamline days, the school turned to television and developed a partnership with four other nursing schools in the Twin Cities. In 1962 Mounds-Midway School of Nursing, Northwestern Hospital School of Nursing, St. Barnabas Hospital School of Nursing, St. Mary's Hospital School of Nursing, and Abbott Hospital School of Nursing formed the Coordinating

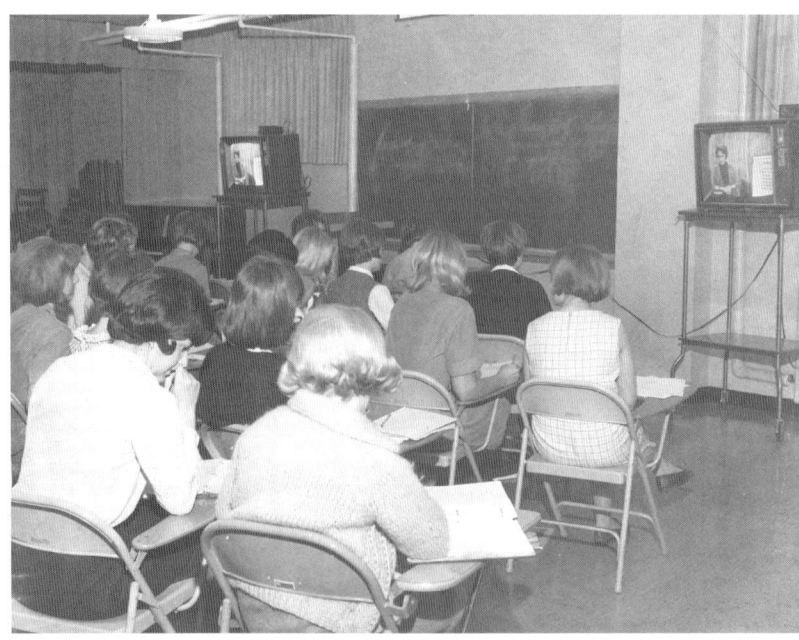

In 1962, Mounds-Midway began providing video classes in the sciences and liberal arts. This photograph is from 1967.

Committee of the Cooperating Schools of KTCA, Video Nursing. This new project in television was a means of providing science courses to all five schools using the same qualified teachers via television. Dr. Lois D. Anderson (1946), who had been educational coordinator at Mounds Park, was the coordinator of the project. She became a passionate advocate for the use of television in nursing education, gaining national recognition for the Twin Cities program.[6]

Courses included anatomy and physiology, communications, pharmacology, sociology (all purchased by Mounds-Midway School of Nursing) and chemistry, microbiology and psychology (which were not purchased). Special instructors from Bethel College taught chemistry and microbiology.[7] Carol Harrison Harms (1971) recalled,

> We had courses on video. I had not been exposed to this type of learning. When you have a typical presentation, in a fifty-minute classroom lecture, the first ten minutes and the last ten are used for introduction and summary, so most of the video lectures were a half-hour. We watched them as a class. You got right to the point with core material. Then, once a week, the instructor came to the school, answered questions, and administered tests. It was helpful to me. I knew that questions wouldn't take the teacher off on a trail that didn't address the core material.

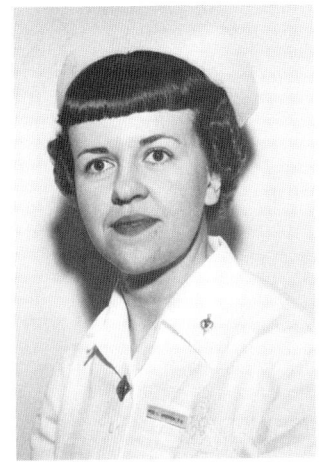

Lois D. Anderson (1946)

The students still gained much of their education through a series of clinical rotations.

Although Mounds Park had been a pioneering psychiatric hospital since its inception, the state began to require that state scholarship students fulfill part of their training at a public institution. This led to an affiliation with Moose Lake State Hospital from 1963 to 1965.

Judy Magnuson Boomer (1965) recalled, "My hardest time was being up in northern Minnesota during the winter rotation. I remember that my roommate and I took the Greyhound bus each weekend back to the Twin Cities, so we wouldn't feel depressed at having to stay indoors, especially during a very tiring time of learning to understand mental health."

Arlys Deckert Schwabauer (1964) remembered the time as a tremendous learning experience:

> The dorm was connected to the hospital by a series of tunnels with pipes, etc. I was always a bit nervous walking through there to the

hospital! One [patient] was always in his long john underwear in an effort to keep him from escaping. He apparently knew all the tricks for getting out! One patient, who was somewhat psychotic, apparently took a dislike to me and threw a marble straight at my eye. Fortunately, I was wearing glasses and no harm was done. I will always remember one thing one of the instructors told us. She said none of us are immune to illnesses as depression, etc. and we should know when we need to get help for ourselves and not consider it shameful.

The experiment was short-lived and psychiatric nursing was returned to the home hospitals in September 1965. However, it was combined with several weeks at Anoka State Hospital.

Pediatrics was still taught at Childrens' Hospital. Carol Hart Brown Harrison (1963) described one memorable experience there. "Carol Klippenstein and I were in the middle of a playroom party for the children," she said. "Several in wheelchairs, the others on the story rug. As leaders watching closely for responses and expressions on the faces of the children, we felt engrossed. After the party, a hospital staff member questioned us sharply about our lack of response to the hospital-wide fire alarm. Carol and I just stared at each other, realizing that we had been so absorbed in the children that we had not even heard the alarm. We apologized, promising to stay more alert, and soon received a top grade for our good party plans."

For many students, the Rural Nursing rotation was a favorite, since it allowed them to get into a small town and the relative freedom of life away from the dorm. Arlys Deckert Schwabauer (1964) described her time at a small hospital in Worthington, Minnesota:

> We lived in a house with students from other hospitals and supplied much of the nursing for the hospital. We were given more responsibility and freedom in our work. We were respected and we worked hard. The community and churches in the area were great to us and included the students in many events. We were there in the fall and celebrated Halloween with a church group.

One key component of that senior year was the team leadership class, another program introduced in 1958. Carol Harrison Harms remembered, "We were taught to work with others, to assign tasks, and to communicate clearly. We assessed who was on the team and what their strengths were: LPNs, RNs, nurses' aides, and around twenty patients. You needed to decide who was best to assign to a particular task and then monitor if they were carried it out."

The Life of a Student Nurse, 1960s

The school continued to draw heavily from the upper Midwest. As an example, in 1962, there were 117 students. Slightly more than half hailed from Minnesota, while Iowa, Wisconsin, and the Dakotas were liberally represented. In terms of religious beliefs, almost two-thirds were Baptist, followed by a contingent of Lutherans, plus a smattering of those from Covenant, Mennonite, Christian and Missionary Alliance, and Presbyterian churches.[8] A survey by the school's Educational Study Committee broke down the primary reasons that students came: 64% selected MMSN for its location, 85% because it was a Christian school, and 64% for its reputation.[9]

No one made a more lasting impact on the students during the sixties than a diminutive woman named Dorothy Lee. When she came to Mounds-Midway in 1959, it was an innovation to have a counselor

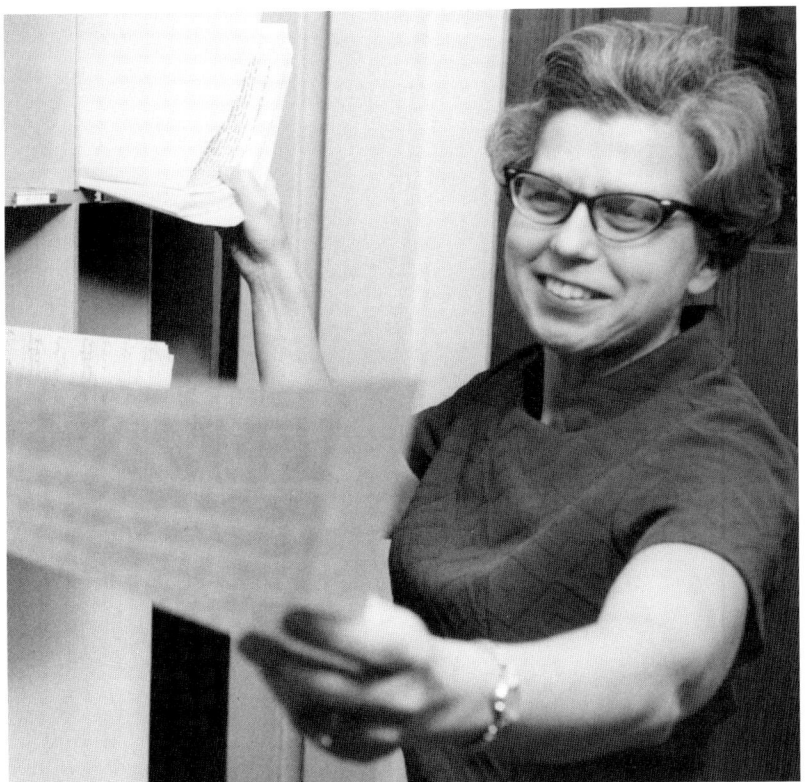

Dorothy Lee

Chapter Four 113

at a diploma school. And, for young women who were brought up being taught, "Jesus first; others second; me, third," Dorothy made them stop and look at themselves. Arlys Deckert Schwabauer (1964) remembered,

> She asked each of us to write an autobiography when we were freshman. She learned a lot about us from this, of course. She was very perceptive. When she realized some of us would need extra support, she was there to give it. I recall crying many tears while I wrote mine, which I'm sure was good for me. Mrs. Lee holds a special place in our hearts. She stood up for us when we needed it and she also helped us understand the times we erred. I suspect she was the best loved faculty person at Mounds-Midway.

Carol Harrison Harms (1971) said that she carried the lessons learned from Dorothy for the rest of her life. "She challenged us to look at who we were," Harms said. "If we are to love God, and our neighbor, as we loved ourselves, then we had to learn about ourselves and love ourselves. This wasn't something selfish. She would tell us, "When we get to heaven, Jesus is not going to ask us, 'Why weren't you Moses?' He will ask, 'Were you the best Carol Harrison that you could be?'

And her influence spread beyond the students. Adella Bennett

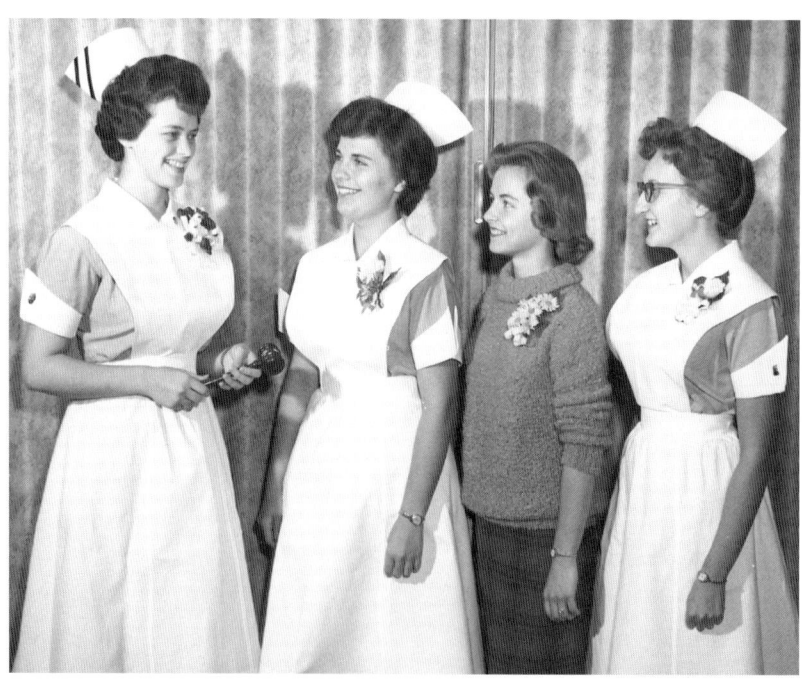

Officers of Women's Association of Mounds-Midway, better known as WAMM. Joanne Muchlow (1962) Sharon Wilford (1963), Diana Waldron (1964), Anne Schoch (1963)

Espelien said, "I loved Dorothy Lee. There is a lot of stress in being a student, dealing with death and dying. It gave the students some place to go. The faculty needed to maintain a distance, because a student should not have to go with personal issues to someone who graded them. We needed it when I was a student. We had no one to talk to about those issues. You kept them inside and that's not healthy. Faculty members often turned to her as well."

With Lee's assistance, Mrs. Sandve empowered the students by creating the Women's Association of Mounds-Midway (WAMM). The organization included representative from each class, the Religious Activities Council, Choir, the *Pre-RN* yearbook, and the Minnesota Nursing Students Association. Together, they sponsored school activities and helped to formulate dorm rules.

The typical progression for housing was that freshmen lived at the Aldine Street dorm, moved up to Mounds Park for their junior year — except for off-campus clinical rotations — then returned to Midway as seniors, usually at the older Shield Street dorm. "This particular dorm was quite an old building that had been renovated for a dorm," wrote Arlys Deckert Schwabauer (1964). "One of the girls woke up with a mouse resting in her hand one morning."

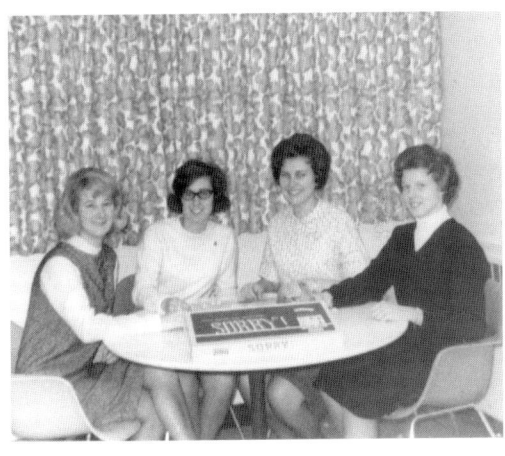

Fun in the dorm, circa 1966. Left to right: Susan Sargeant Buelow, Jan Heida Dexter, Karen Smit Veninga, Kathleen Shaw Brandt (all 1967).

The stress of dorm life and long hours demanded a release. Food, of course, happened to be one of the outlets. Arlys Deckert Schwabauer (1964) recalled, "I was rooming with Carol Radke Kejr (1964) and her family had sent a care package with a couple of cans of lemonade concentrate. We didn't refrigerate it. For some reason, it exploded one night after we'd gone to bed and it bounced around the room a few times before coming to rest." Bonnie Erichsen Scherer fondly recalled, "Bologna, mustard and pickle sandwiches made and eaten in the dorm because cafeteria food was not what it was cracked up to be."

Whenever the pressure of exams and work threatened to overwhelm the students, there was always Mrs. Chase to relieve the tension. Paula Willie remembered, "We had a couple mannequins in the resource center and I would sneak down and take one of them up to the room of someone who was out for the evening. They would come home and see someone sitting in their room."

Chapter Four 115

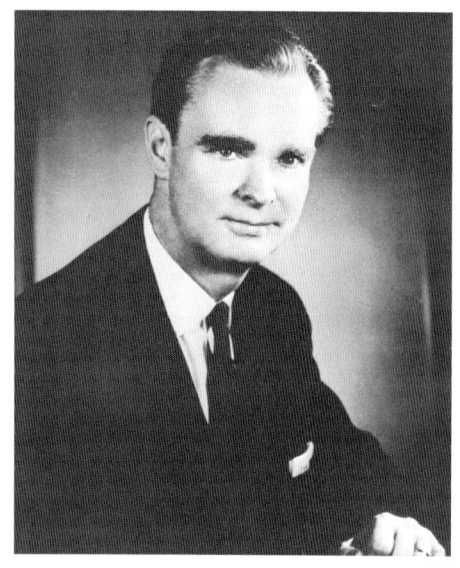

The Singer's Prayer

*Take Thou my lips, dear Lord,
and may I sing Thy message clearly.
Take Thou my heart and mind,
and may I sing my song sincerely.
O take my lips, my heart, my mind,
And when I've sung, O let me find
That some soul through me
Has been led unto Thee.
This is Thy servant's prayer.*

James P. Davies

Above: James Davies, Choir director

Right: The "Now Sound" of the Choir. Left to right: Lilyan Renaud Eliason (1970), Faith Rich (1971), Sue Ohmann Groff (1971), Janet Chatfield Wachter (1970).

Below: The Choir embarks on a tour to Michigan in 1965.

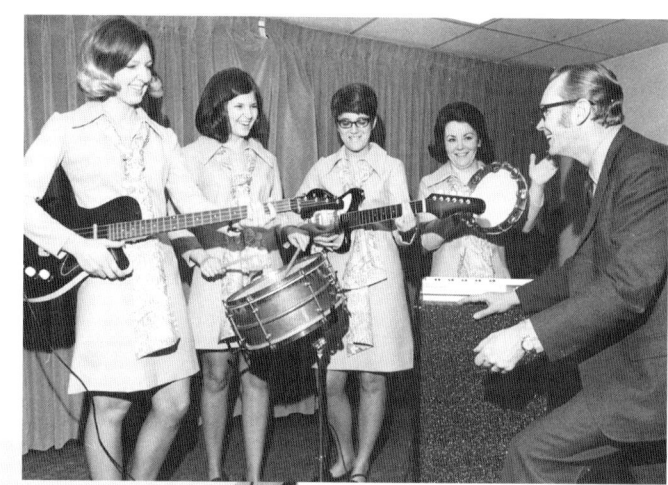

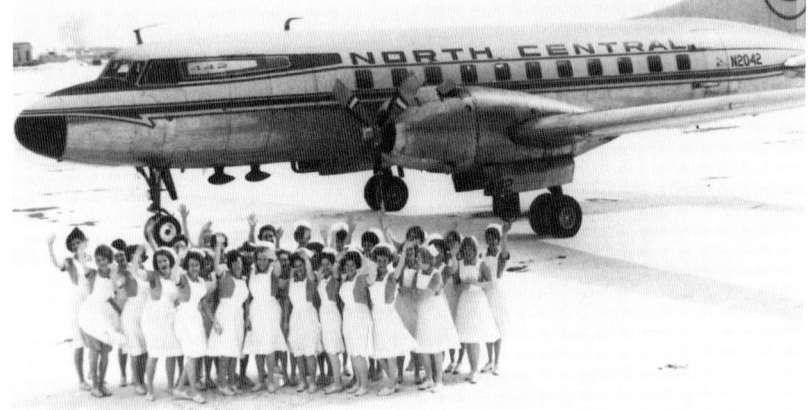

A Singer's Prayer

"Singing in the choir was a highlight of my student days," Judy Webster McCrory (1965) wrote. The feeling was shared by many of those who sat under the leadership of Jim Davies during the sixties and seventies. A talented director, Davies had founded the Moody Chorale before coming to Mounds-Midway and wrote a book for choirs entitled, *Sing . . . With Understanding*—a title that suggests his special gift. Lilyan Renaud Eliason summarized his impact, saying, "Jim Davies was a spiritual mentor as well as a talented director."[10]

Practice and concerts were memorable for the opportunity to sing, but also because of the spiritual emphasis. Judy Magnuson Boomer (1965) recalled, "We traveled all over, singing mostly in churches, and staying in the homes of people. Our director always provided a time at the end of each concert which he called 'the redeemed of the Lord say so.' It was a time when nurses shared their personal thoughts after our songs. I felt that our travels certainly promoted the profession of nursing. I felt we were respected, and at the same time, showed them our human side representing God's love. Sharing time with the other gals gave us a closeness during our training."

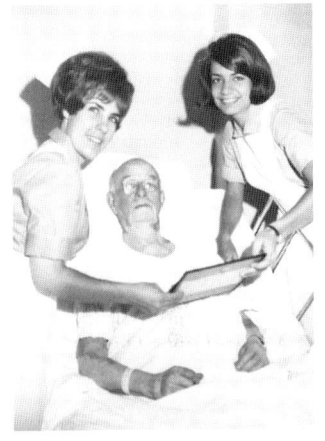

While a patient, John Jaeger, longtime choir director, received special care from Anita Smith Erickson and Eunice Anderson in 1967.

The best evidence of Davies's insistence on musical excellence was the occasional competition that the choir entered. Picture a warm August night along the shores of Lake Michigan in 1962. On that evening, fifty-two thousand people gathered in Soldiers Field for the annual Chicagoland Music Festival. The *Chicago Tribune* described it as "a thrilling spectacle. It was the county fair, an old-time songfest, a tent revival, an evening in the park, all of these great things of the past and present rolled into one." The evening's stars included opera star Robert Merrill, comedian Phyllis Diller, and a popular composer and singer named Ned Washington, who was coaxed by the audience to sing his Academy Award-winning hit, "When You Wish Upon A Star." Then came performances by the music competition winners—among them, the first place women's choir from the Mounds-Midway School of Nursing singing "Old Joe Clark." It was, said the *Tribune*, "a fine moment for the show." Bonnie Erichsen Scherer (1962) remembered, "It was overwhelming for this South Dakota girl!"[11]

"Directing a nurses' choir isn't as easy as it looks, Davies said. "It's the only group I've ever led where it was virtually impossible to have all members present at the same time for rehearsals." Still, he found the time to begin a handbell choir and to take the choir into the recording studio on several occasions.[12]

Chapter Four   117

The first Lucia Festival, 1958. Left to right: Carol Ann Edminister, Jeanette Bibelheimer, Ulla Tervonen, Waynce Sandve, Judy Anderson

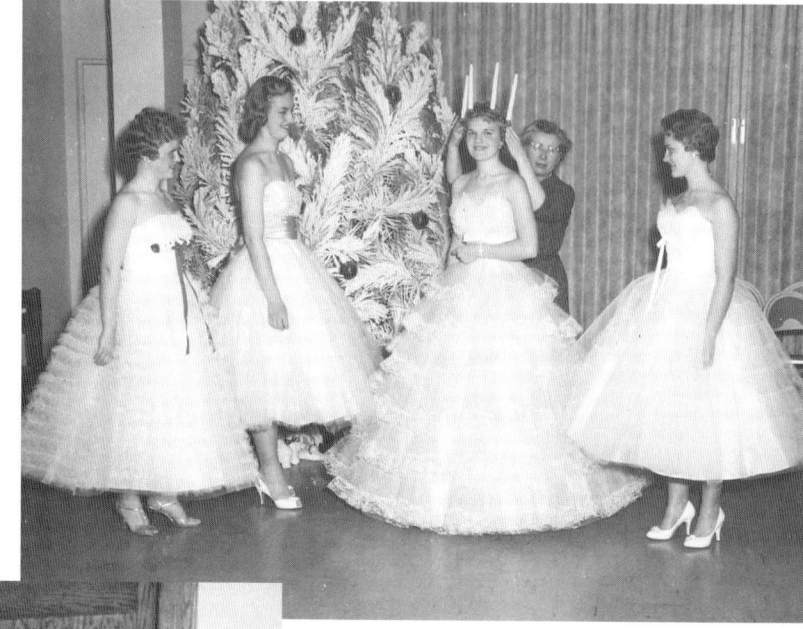

Stripe Day, 1963

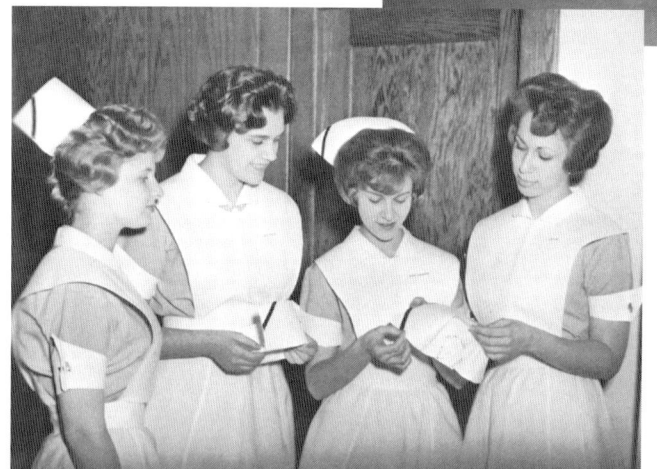

Annette Grandin with Carol Erickson Kalmbacher, at graduation, 1967. Grandin remained an important link to the past, retiring in 1974 after thirty-seven years.

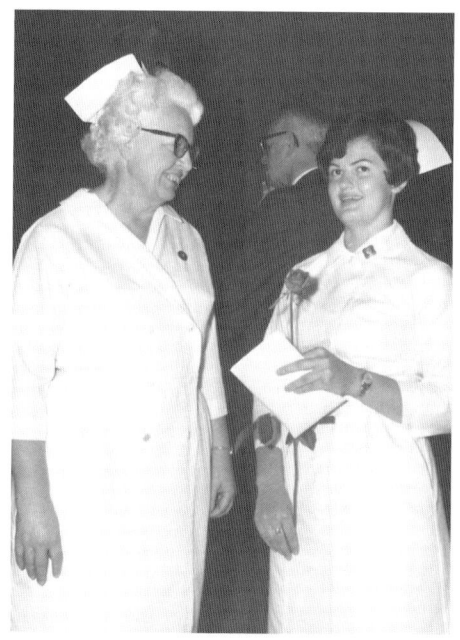

Sandve recognized the importance of rituals to bring the school together, reporting to the state nursing board, "We are in the process of establishing new traditions and reviving activities for the whole student group." With that in mind, she reached back to the school's Swedish heritage and began an annual Santa Lucia Day. Freshmen chose the honoree as "one who typifies the Christmas spirit of giving and spreading joy and happiness."

Capping remained an important event. Judy Magnuson Boomer was asked to share her personal thoughts as part of her capping service. "I remember saying," Boomer wrote, That my cap would give me a chance to share my love for God, and used the C-Christ, A-Approaches, P-Patients as a description in my talk. I felt that by choosing this profession, I would be able to reach out to help others, not only physically (in giving them comfort) but also emotionally (in giving them a listening ear, and a compassionate touch)."

Myrna Kern Opp (1965) was also asked to speak at her class ceremony, held at Central Baptist Church. However, the capping in her junior year proved to be even more memorable.

> As a junior I presented a cap to my little sis in the freshman class. It was because of this event that I met my husband. Don, my husband to be, attended this ceremony as a date with one of the freshman student nurses and took notice of a few of the other student nurses there. He was able to get the names from the name tags on our uniforms and made a list of possible prospective dates. My name was on the list. Sometime later I received a phone call from this gentleman asking me to go on a date. It was a blind date for me but not for him. We began dating and were married the next June after my graduation from MMSN.

Opp noted, "We celebrated our forty-first wedding anniversary in June 2006."

The march toward graduation that began with capping would be marked by other events. These included Stripe Day, when juniors received their first stripe and seniors their second, and Halfway and Two-thirds parties to mark the student's progress toward graduation.

As graduation approached, seniors shared a tradition on the last day on the floors. Arlys Deckert Schwabauer described Ripping Day: "Their uniforms were cut and some of the young women came back to the dorm with their clothing in shreds! No one was upset by it, of course. I have a picture of this somewhere. My grandmother made a quilt of my blue and white student uniforms. I don't believe I have it anymore. I wore it out."

Graduation was still "a big deal" as several graduates claimed. "We were real nurses!" No commencement address had more of an immediate impact than one given to the graduating class of 1965 by Dr. Robert Hingson, a Christian physician and professor of anesthesiology at Western Reserve University. He challenged the graduates to consider joining him in Honduras over the summer. Judy Webster McCrory (1965), with the support of her parents, volunteered, joined by three classmates. She wrote later, "It made our hearts ache to see the small emaciated bodies, so full of worms, so undernourished, and nearly everyone with diarrhea. There is lots of impetigo and I became expert in giving baths, cutting hair, and covering little bodies oozing with sores using our only medicine, some bactine. We treated dog bites, infected feet, and numerous other sores."

The school, under the guidance of the Baptist Hospital Fund, continued to place a strong emphasis on the spiritual development of the students. Students now took religion courses each year. Although attendance at morning chapel was now voluntary, attendance remained strong. In addition, students gathered at weekly convocations, featuring special speakers and programs on educational, professional, and

Adella Bennett Espelien, director, 1964-1966

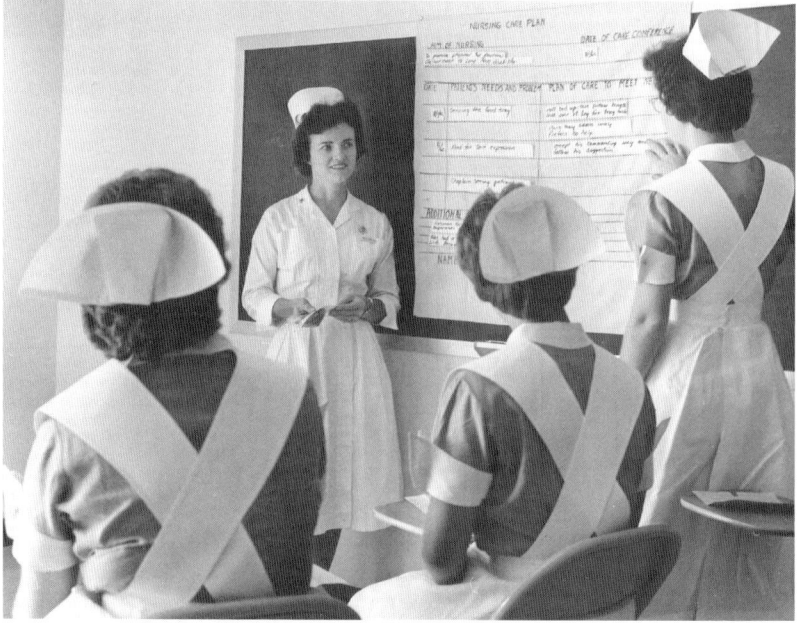

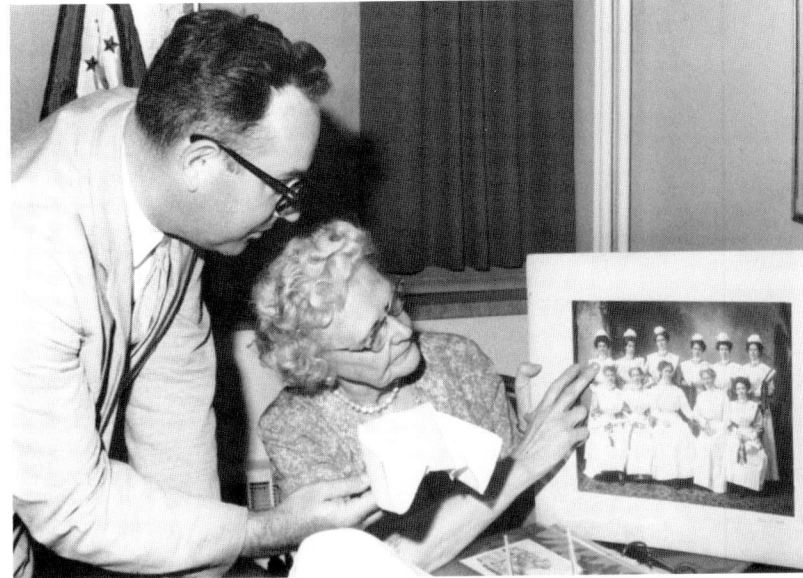

Ruth Gustafson shows a historic photograph to Gordon Smith, director of development and education for the Baptist Hospital Fund.

religious subjects. Many were active in Nurses' Christian Fellowship and the Religious Council organized a Deeper Life Week every year.

Judy Magnuson Boomer (1965) recalled, "I feel that the spiritual growth during my years at Mounds-Midway, has continued to strengthen me in my personal life, and profession life. It prepared me for the many challenges I would face in the future. Not only was a I getting an education, but I was made to feel that I mattered, and I could make a difference in the lives who would come across my path."

Others, such as Judy Kempton Peter (1962) struggled with the spiritual atmosphere. "I found much of the religiosity negative," she said. "The type of religion I saw at Mounds-Midway among the students was often self-serving and condemning of others who did not believe as they did. I was raised as a clergyman's daughter and my upbringing was much more open to others."

Changes

During these years, the Mounds-Midway School of Nursing was responsible to the Board of Trustees of the Baptist Hospital Fund. From 1958 to 1964 the director of the school was directly responsible to the School of Nursing Committee, a subcommittee of the Board of Trustees. During 1964-1966 the organizational chart was changed so that the director of the School of Nursing was directly responsible to the executive director of the Baptist Hospital Fund, Inc., Mel Conley, and through him to the School of Nursing Committee.

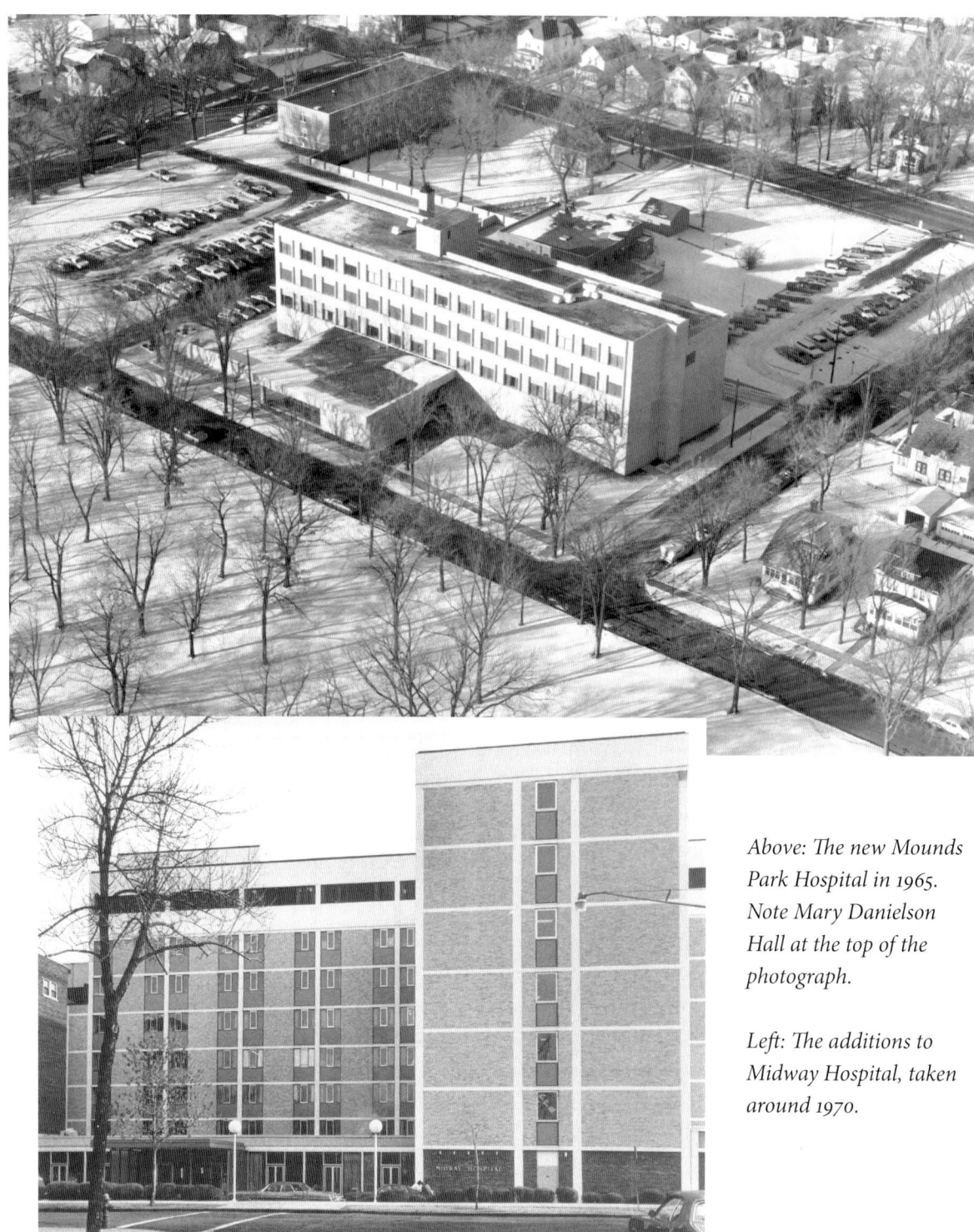

Above: The new Mounds Park Hospital in 1965. Note Mary Danielson Hall at the top of the photograph.

Left: The additions to Midway Hospital, taken around 1970.

In 1964, Sandve decided to accept a teaching position at Gustavus Adolphus College. The board searched for a replacement for several months, finally deciding to stay with a respected faculty member and MMSN graduate, Adella Bennett Espelien. Committed to high academic standards, Espelien instituted a thorough review of the school, working with a board-appointed Educational Study Committee. Its report was completed in February 1966.

Judy Magnuson Boomer sensed that Espelien "represented our profession at its highest. She always wanted the best for us and expected us to be the best representative of Mounds-Midway that we could be. She was kind and very reachable if we needed help of any kind."

The school gained another strong advocate when Rev. Gordon Smith was hired by the Baptist Hospital Fund as director of development in 1963, with his responsibility growing in 1966 to include general supervision of the educational programs of the Fund, including the School of Nursing.

There were other major changes taking place that radically transformed the two hospitals. In 1965, the old Mounds Park Hospital was demolished to make way for a completely new 136-bed facility. At the dedication ceremonies, Dr. George Earl announced that the dormitory would be named after Mary Danielson. By the end of the sixties, the hospital added fourth and fifth floors, bringing capacity of the hospital to 216 beds. Meanwhile, at Midway, the old hospital had a major addition in 1962, adding 124 beds at a cost of $3,350,000. As with Mounds Park, the expansion continued with another addition by 1969, bringing its capacity to 337 beds.[13]

Adella Espelien, working with the board, continued to explore long-range options for the school. Diploma schools were increasingly under attack from professional organizations. For example, the American Nurses Association, in a 1965 position paper, stated: "Education for all those who are licensed to practice nursing should take place in the institutions of higher education." So it was clear to Espelien and others that a transition to a collegiate program was necessary. the planning committee reviewed several proposals, including the establishment of an independent Mounds-Midway College of Nursing. A renewed appeal to Bethel College fell on deaf ears, since "Bethel College is moving way out to Arden Hills, and is not particularly interested in a nursing program in the near future."

Remembering those days, Espelien said, "We started trying to figure out what to do. We investigated a relationship with Bethel. Then the

Chapter Four

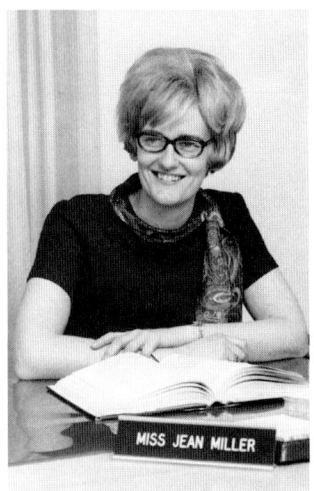

Jean Miller, director from 1966 to 1968

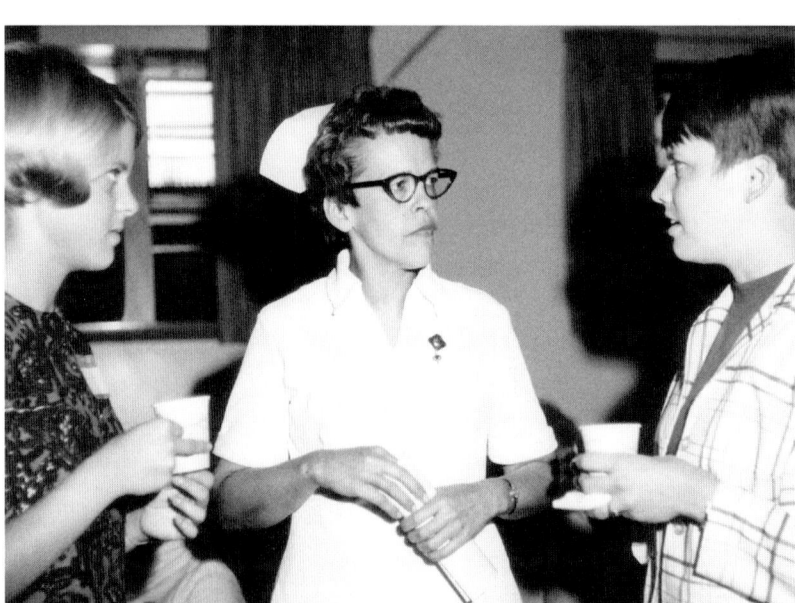

Virginia Anderson, director from 1968 to 1971

board said to look at Sioux Falls College." In 1965, serious discussions began with Sioux Falls (South Dakota) College aimed at a complete merger of the school of nursing into that Baptist institution. The ties were strong—influential Baptist Hospital Fund board member Norman Mears was also chairman of the Sioux Falls College Board of Trustees. Chester Stone and Dr. Clifford Perron also sat on both boards.[14]

Negotiations advanced so far that Mel Conley reported: "The plans for the proposed baccalaureate program in cooperation with Sioux Falls College are still not complete, however, tentative approval has been given by both boards." Indeed, when Mrs. Espelien resigned in 1966 to follow her physician husband to Saint Cloud, the board turned to Jean Miller as an interim director for the upcoming school year, since "by that time, the plans with Sioux Falls College should be finalized." However, concerns about cross-state nursing boards and the distance between the campuses killed the merger in the eleventh-hour of negotiations.

With the collapse of these plans, Jean Miller lost the "interim" part of her title. She was a graduate of the University of Minnesota, with a B. S. and a Masters of Nursing, she had served on the faculty in Med/Surg from 1963 to 1966. Karen Smit Veninga (1967) said that Miller was "more laid back" than her predecessor. "She would tell me to remember that my play was as important as my work."

With strong academic credentials, she pressed to implement the

124   THIS CAP OF WHITE

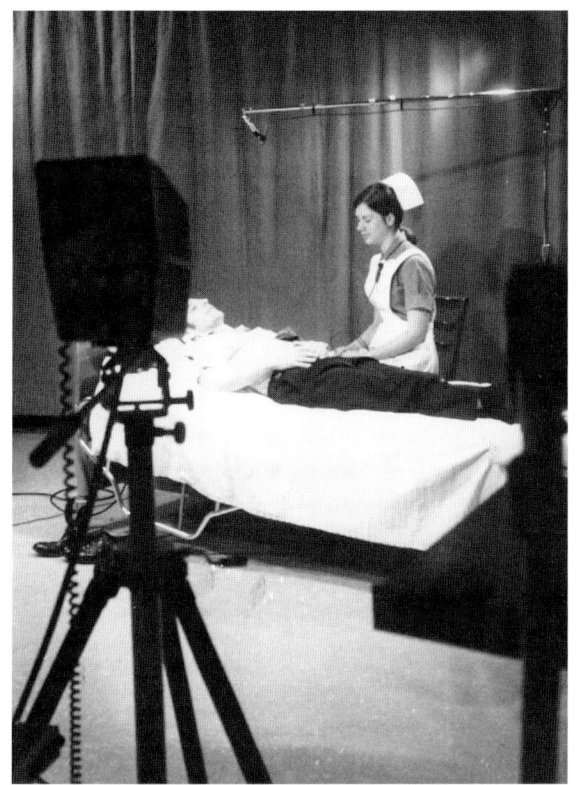

Mounds-Midway received a major grant to develop its Learning Resource Center (below), including a television studio (left). Curtis Johnson (below) was hired to direct the program, becoming the school's first full-time male faculty member.

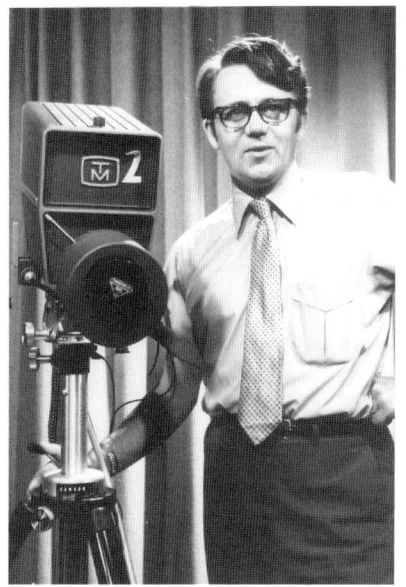

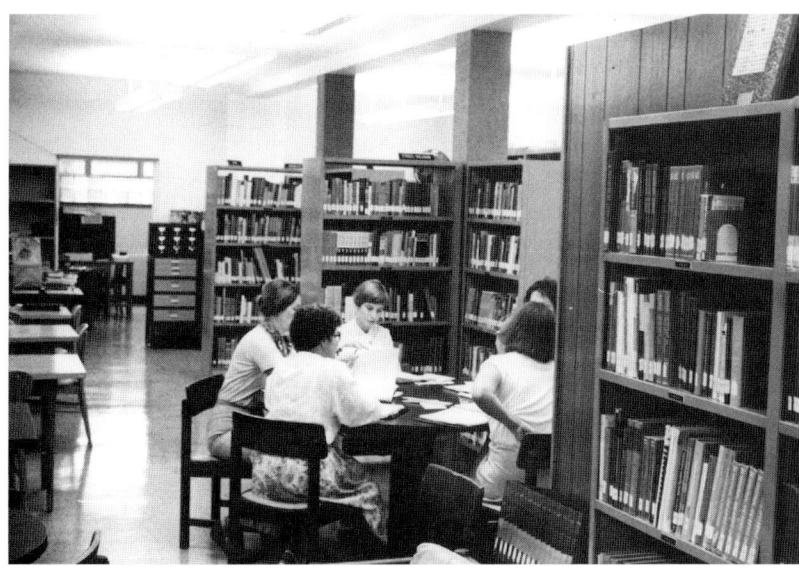

The new Learning Resource Center also included materials for the new audio-tutorial teaching method. Below: Delores Martin reviews a slide program.

Lorraine Lilja

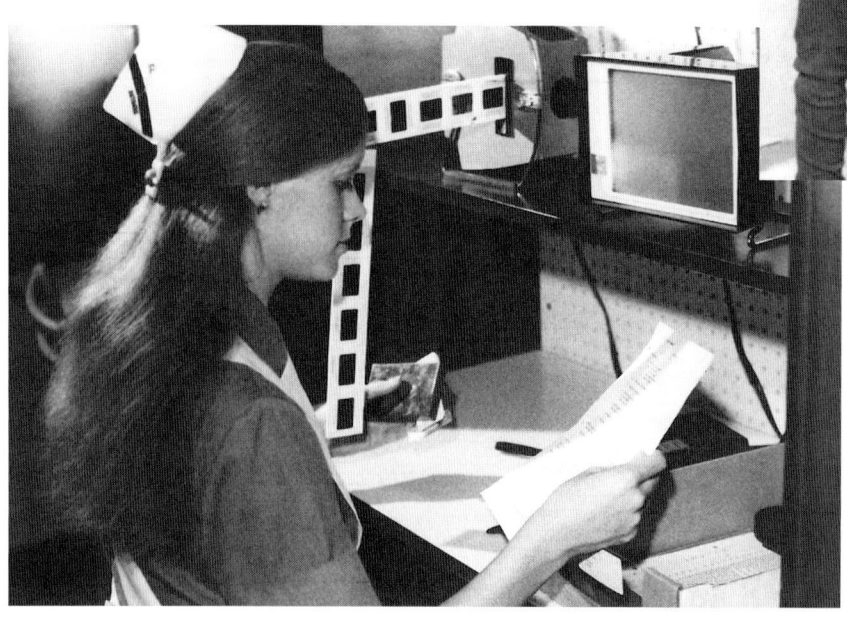

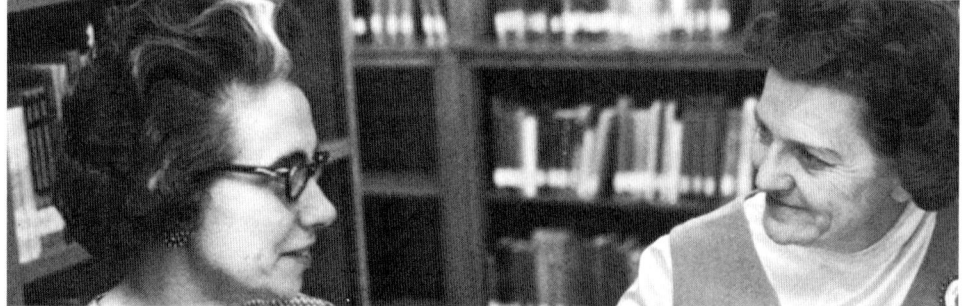

Librarians Carol Windham (left) and Emily Halversen (right).

recommendations of the self-study, leading to the award of a substantial grant from the federal government in 1969 to establish an audio-tutorial educational program. However, Miller's heart was set on furthering her education and, as she said, "It would become too comfortable if I remained too long as director." Following her passion, she left in 1968 to pursue first a M.A. and then a Ph.D. in sociology from the University of Washington. She resumed her teaching career, eventually serving on the faculty at the University of Rhode Island. As the Weyker Endowed Chair in Thanology, she initiated a post-baccalaureate program on issues of death and dying.

She was followed by Virginia Anderson, a 1948 graduate of Mounds-Midway and longtime clinical instructor. After leaving the hospital in 1960 to pursue a master's degree in nursing administration, she became director of nursing services at Shriners Hospital in Minneapolis and then spent four years as occupational health nurse at General Mills.

One of Anderson's principal contributions was the implementation of the new audio-tutorial instructional program, hiring the first full-time male faculty member, Curtis Johnson. A Bethel graduate, he had been editor of *Impact*, an American Baptist magazine, and had formerly been a pastor. Under his guidance, the audio-tutorial method became a key component of the curriculum for the next decade. Looking back on the program, Beth Peterson (1971) reflected, "There was a strong expectation that students would use the lab and library to prepare for class and clinical. We also had staff in place that made that possible — Emily Halverson, Lorraine Lilja, Curt Johnson. There was a real emphasis on thinking and learning, not on rote memorization or 'doing what we were told to do.' I had no trouble making the shift to a baccalaureate nursing program."

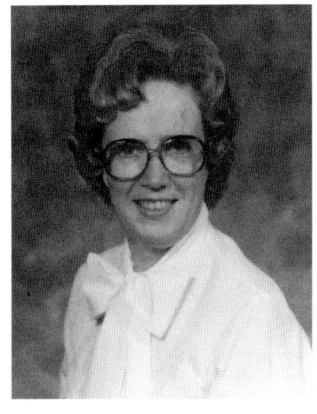

Charlotte Sandin Olson, director, 1971 to 1983

Anderson also initiated a curriculum revision. Carol Harrison Harms (1971) served as student representative on the committee during her senior year. Recalling with pleasure the opportunity to work with dedicated faculty members, she said, "We asked 'What are our goals?' We decided to build the curriculum around the concept of optimal health — what was the best that could be achieved for each patient. For example, if a someone has cerebral palsy, what is optimal health for that person? The patient is not going to run the marathon, but what obstacles can be addressed?"

The revision was completed and implemented by yet another director, Charlotte Sandin Olson. Olson had worked at Mounds-Midway, off and on, for nearly two decades when she stepped into the director's

Chapter Four

position. She ushered in a period of relative stability, remaining as director for longer than any other except Mary Danielson. With her staff, Olson implemented the new teaching concept called "Optimal Health." She explained the philosophy:

> Beginning with the concept of optimal health and the basic need of the individual throughout his/her developmental growth, and based on concepts of homeostasis and adaptation, the student moves to deviations from the normal with emphasis through the whole program of adapting to the anomalies and the situation in order to maintain whatever is optimal health for any individual.

Evaluating "Optimal Health" from her perspective as a teacher, Elizabeth Peterson said, "Looking back, I realize how revolutionary that idea was. Most diploma schools focused on illness issues, but I think faculty bought into a much broader philosophy of what nursing could and should be and kept it alive. Structures were in place to continue the 'spirit' of the curriculum revision right up until the school closed."

Enrollment reached an all-time high as well. In 1973, there were 181 students enrolled, including a freshman class of seventy-four members.

The Education of a Nurse, 1970s

In this decade, students began their freshman year at Midway

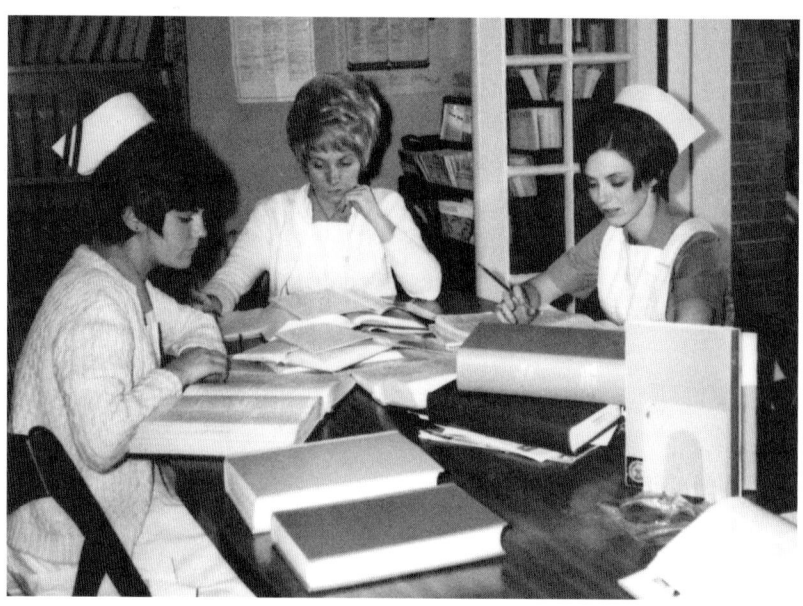

Working on a care plan at the Children's Hospital library, December 1969. Left to right: Lenny Gustafson, Janice Roth, and Carol Parker.

Hospital, where they took science classes and Nursing 101 — an update of the old Fundamentals of Nursing course. During the second year, juniors moved to Mounds Park and broke into smaller groups for clinicals. Connie Dreyer (1975) fondly remembered the casual atmosphere at Mounds during her junior year: "I thought they were a group of nurses that were warm, compassionate and caring. Mounds was like a family and there seemed to be more of a neighborhood connection. It was, we would say now, a little lower tech." Then, for the final year, they returned to Midway.

Although the courses were regularly fine-tuned, the 1977 course list gives us a snapshot of the typical student schedule in the last decade of the school.

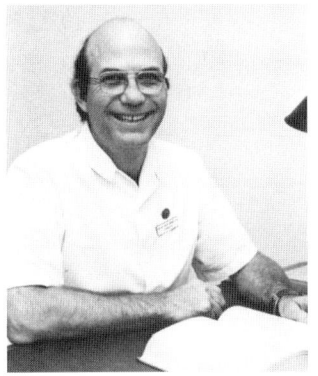

Brother Joseph Warnert

Freshmen
   Chemistry of Life Processes
   Anatomy and Physiology
   Religion I
   Interpersonal Competencies
   Nursing 101
   Literary Forms
   Microbiology and Parasitology
   Introduction to Psychology
   Nutrition
   Nursing 102

Junior
   Pharmacology I and II
   Diet Therapy
   Nursing 201
   Religion II
   Sociology
   Nursing 202
   Human Development
   Nursing 203

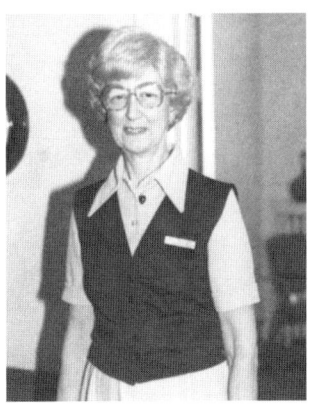

Florence Olson

Senior
   Man and Morality
   Nursing 301, 302, 303, 304
   Fine Arts
   Family Life

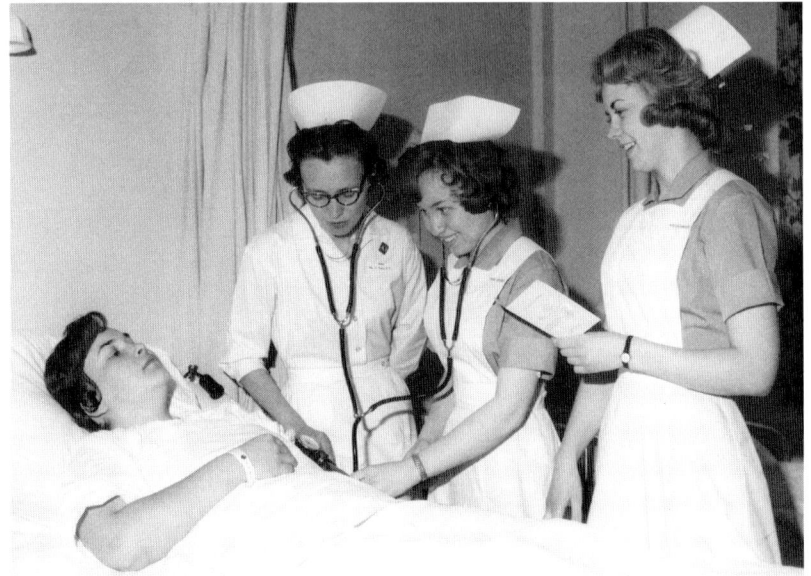

Left to right: "Patient" Judy Stegmeier, Instructor Gladys Benson Karhu (1951), Jan Bloomquist, and Lois Jefson

The techniques included, in the first half of the decade, continued use of television instruction, plus use of audio tapes and self-study learning modules. Under Curtis Johnson and Lorraine Lilja, with assistance from librarians Emily Halvorsen and Carol Windham, the audio-visual prograam developed an outstanding learning resource center, opened in 1971 on the lower level of the Midway dormitory. It included the library, an audio-visual lab, and a television studio.

The curriculum now employed on a more holistic approach, helping the student focus on the patient. Pam Ruberto-Krugman (1976) wrote about "three priceless practices" that she learned.

- At bedtime we were asked to get into bed and without adjusting for comfort, stay in that initial position for one hour. That exercise was to teach us that turning our patients every hour was not only necessary but a long time for them to wait for us.
- We were required for one day, to be blind-folded and be led around by our partner. The next day we reversed roles. The purpose of this lesson was two-fold: to teach us to anticipate our patients' needs, and to understand being disabled.
- We were trained to chart precisely and acurately for possible litigation. Because of this training, my charting was given exemplary honor for terminating litigation twice.

The psych rotation continued to both shock and fascinate the students. Paula Willie recalled, "Psych scared me. My first patient was a nurse and she kept telling me that her problems all started when she was in nursing school. Always disturbing to hear!"

One teacher who made a major impact was Brother Joseph Warnert, instructor in Psychiatric Nursing from 1973 to 1978. A pioneer, Warnert was the first male student at St. Catherine's and the first Christian Brother in the history of the order to earn a nursing degree. Connie Dreyer reminisced, "Brother Joe Warnert was good. He asked us what we felt least comfortable with. I said young people and probably young men. So he assigned me a young man. I remember the whole time in clinical with this young guy."

One major change was addition of a psychiatric rotation at Veterans' Hospital in Minneapolis. Here, students worked with older men suffering neurological disorders. For example, one student recalled a bright former professor suffering from aphasia. "He would ask to have the blinds open, when he meant shut. I cannot imagine how frustrating it must have been for him." Florence Olson taught the course.

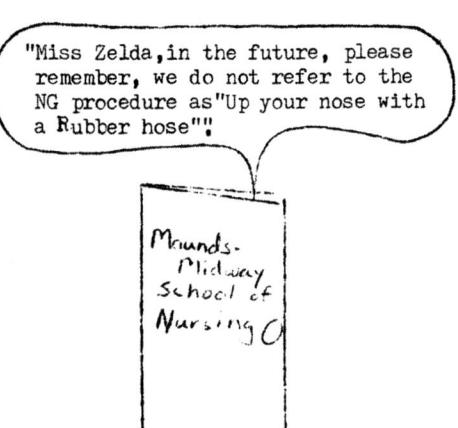

From the student newspaper, The Sternum Star, 1980

Another well-loved instructor, Gladys Benson Karhu (1951), began teaching surgery at MMSN in the early sixties. She was, one student wrote, "a thorough nurse, who expects her students to continually broaden their field of knowledge. One essential skill that we have learned from this caring nurse is to communicate through touch. Frequently she expresses concern to those around her by giving an encouraging pat or an emphatic hand squeeze." Another recalled how Karhu would come by and "put her cold hands on the back of your neck so that you wouldn't pass out when it got so hot."

Lois Bernhardson, who taught junior nursing clinicals between 1973 and 1983, was remembered by one student as "no nonsense but fair. She was older and real comfortable with herself." Bernhardson collected student uniforms, eventually made into a quilt with more than 3,000 pieces. It helped, she said, to recall her years with "great young people."

There were difficult lessons in suffering, pain, and death to be learned. Cheryl McBride Dietrich (1970) remembered a stressful introduction to Obstetrics: "The first delivery I saw was a fetus with an IUD in its head. I went back to the dorm and went under the covers. My clinical instructor came over and spoke with me.... I got the rest of the day off but the next day I was back at OB clinical."

Paula Willie said, "This patient — I was working nights — had trouble breathing so I sat his bed up and he was much better. I had stepped out of the room for a while when an aide came and asked, 'Is the guy in nineteen supposed to be dead?' I didn't know. I don't remember what he came in for and his death wasn't expected."

Still, there were light moments. One student nurse wrote,

> My most embarrassing moment was when I was a junior working in the OR recovery room. I volunteered to take a cystoscopy patient back to the short stay area. I was recklessly driving the cart down the hall to the elevator. No one was around to help me hold the elevator door while pushing the cart into it. During the process I got my hair caught on the hook of the IV pole. So here I am trying to unhook my hair, hoping and praying that no one would come and use the elevator. Except the patient could see me — quite embarrassing. I managed to unhang myself by ripping my hair out and proceeded to fix my hair to look presentable.[15]

Alys DuCharme, who was a faculty member from 1972 to 1975, and again from 1978 to 1982, summarized her feelings about those years:

> What stands out is the sense of camaraderie that existed between faculty, students, and hospital staff. I always felt that no matter what was going on in our lives and our world, things were solid, grounded, and leading towards common goals at MMSN. Of course there were serious moments of thoughtful discussion, and sometimes discipline, but we did things prayerfully, knowing that we weren't alone.

Naomi Smith, who served on the faculty from 1977 to 1981, echoed these thoughts, stating: "It was a supportive, accepting, caring and stimulating atmosphere, and that is rare in groups today. I did look forward to going to work, interacting and laughing with my colleagues. They became real friends."

The Life of a Student Nurse, 1970s

Student life reflected the changes of American society of the late sixties and seventies. Students no longer quietly accepted the admin-

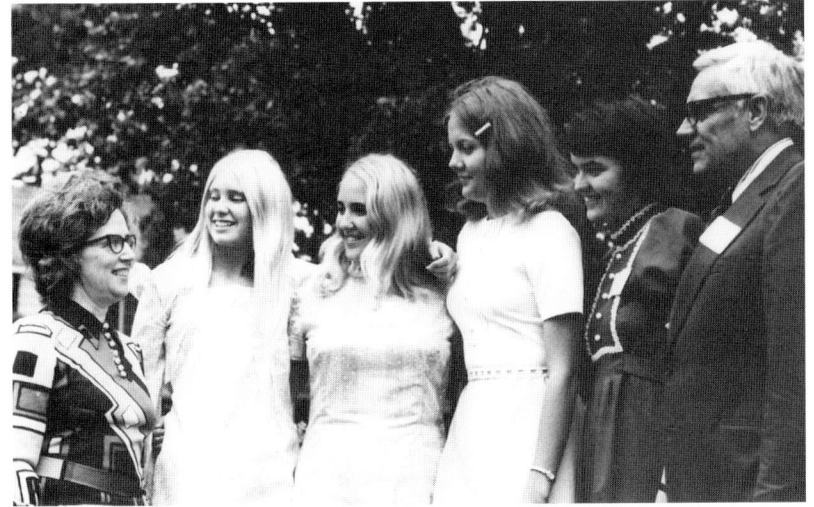

Charlotte Olson (left) and her husband, Mike (right) greet new students in the fall of 1972. Left to right: Sheri Gilquist Miller, Valerie Miller, Marilyn Olson Schreiber, Colleen Dewing Sugimoto

istration and faculty rules and regulations. In 1970, there was even a minor rebellion, as Virginia Anderson noted in her annual report to the state nursing board:

> There has been some student unrest, which came out in the open following the discipline of four students for drinking. As a result of this, the students have met with the faculty and in student-faculty committees. The students have requested some changes and want individual and committee responsibilities, as they relate to extracurricular activities, to be more clearly defined so they know where everyone stands.

As Carol Harrison Harms said, "We were movers and shakers and if we saw something and we didn't see a good reason, we would question it, I think, in a fairly respectable way. We would go as a group to Mel Conley or Gordon Smith and say, we want this to change." Elizabeth Peterson recalled the how, with the help of Dorothy Lee, students organized a day to discuss the Vietnam War, with speakers offering different perspectives.

Student life also changed as the doors opened to new applicants. Older married women were now welcomed. For example, Mary Fischbach (1980) had worked as an x-ray technician in the 1950s, then turned to raising her two children. As they grew up, she decided that "volunteering and playing bridge" was not for her, so she entered Mounds-Midway School of Nursing. It was, she said, "a big challenge" but had "a lot of personal satisfaction." Classmate Bonnie LaPanta (1980) had

Chapter Four 133

a similar experience. After a difficult hospital stay following surgery, she related the experience to her prayer group, prompting one of her friends to ask, "Since you feel so strongly, why don't you go out and be a nurse?" With encouragement from her husband and teenage children, she went first to community college and then Mounds-Midway. She was even elected president of the junior class!

The admission of men brought a new dynamic to the school. What should they wear? The men's uniform included white trousers and blue shirt, white socks, and white shoes, but no cap. With so much of the program geared to women, some changes had to be made. WAMM became SAMM — Students Association of Mounds-Midway. The first male student was Allen Butkowski, a transfer, followed by Stephen Trost.

The change was generally taken in stride. Mike Monzel, who graduated in 1980, found that "the instructors were very impartial." Monzel illustrates that the addition of men brought fresh perspective to Mounds-Midway, since he had worked for seven years with a private ambulance service and his wife was a nurse. These were scarcely radicals, although they were breaking gender barriers. As Trost noted, "I have very fond memories of MMSN and to this day still wear my school pin when I wear any type of uniform. I am one of the last nurses who still wears a pin where I work."

Men, however, did not live in the dormitories, and, indeed, increas-

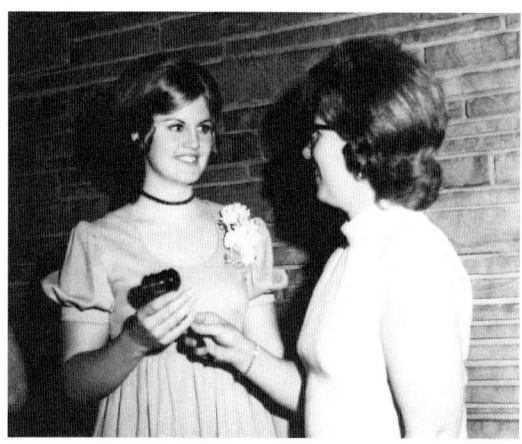

Honors Day, 1972

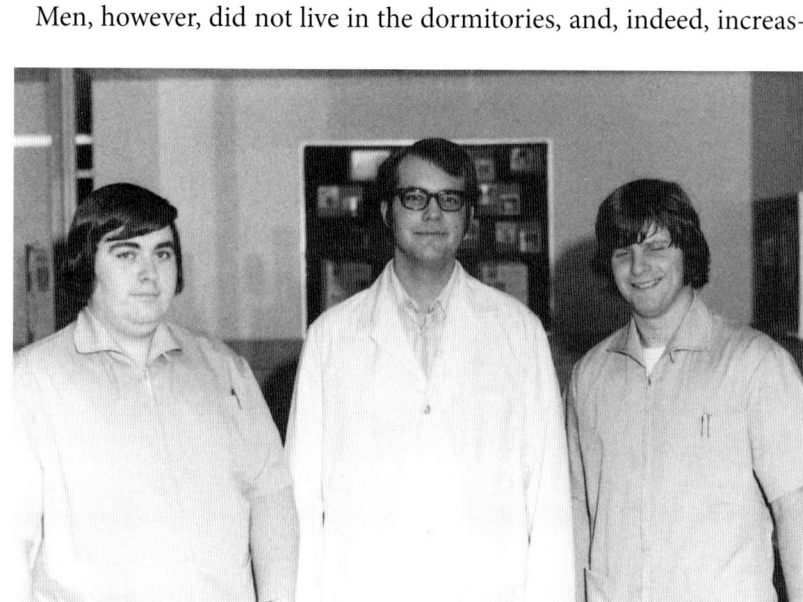

Men were admitted for the first time in 1972. Left to right: Stephen Trost, Allen Butkowski, Jim Bauer.

ing numbers of students lived off-campus. After 1977, Mary Danielson Hall was no longer used as a dormitory. Still, the typical student shared life on Aldine Street. Bev Desens Case (1982) fondly recalled, "Together we discovered the best places to eat. Together, we dieted, snacked, and feasted. Together, we found the best places to shop and found the best bargains around. Together, we studied for IQS, IPC, Chemistry, Anatomy, and Religion. Together, we cried over the bad times and together we laughed over the good times."

Many remembered the "house moms." "They were so great," said Kris Swanson Yard (1976). "For many of us this was our first time away from home and it was so nice to always be greeted by a friendly face. I still laugh about one of the 'mom's' that answered a phone call for me and told my friend that "Kris is overeating" — meaning that I was having dinner at the hospital across the street. So, I was over eating, not overeating. If you remember hospital food, you know I certainly was not 'overeating!'"

And the "moms" kept an eye on you as well, added Swanson. "Looking back on it, I see fun times but things were a bit frustrating at the time. I remember once being about 2 minutes late for curfew and actually getting some sort of 'house arrest'. It wasn't called that but I had to stay in my room without phone calls or being able to leave."

The prospect of romance still distracted many young students from their studies. Paula Willie said that although "there wasn't much dating," an engagement led to a ritual unique to the later classes — the ring-down. A student who was engaged would return to the dorm and tell the R.A. Another student described the occasion:

> Someone would run down the hall in the dorm yelling "ring down, ring down" and everyone would gather in the hallway. There would be a long tapered candle with a diamond ring around the bottom. It would be lit and passed from person to person. When the person who had become engaged got the candle, they would blow it out and everyone would scream their congratulations!

Choir

Choir, still under the baton of Jim Davies, remained special. The music now included more popular tunes by Christian composers such as Ralph Carmichael or Ken Medema, often accompanied by guitars and a tambourine. Describing this new direction, Susan Ackerman said, "It is our attempt to bridge the generation gap by incorporating the Now Sound of amplified guitars and percussion instruments into our concert of traditional sacred music and by the use of visual aids to touch all the senses." The sense of sight was enhanced, during the early seventies, by accompanying multimedia presentations by Curtis Johnson. The music continued to be a worship experience for the churches where they performed and a marketing tool for prospective students and financial support.

For its members, it was a time to enjoy beautiful music and to learn from the shared experiences. Of course, the high point of each year was the tour. Lilyan Renaud Eliason said, "The bus trip to the Dakotas and Minnesota during my senior year was rewarding due to the quality of the program that we presented night after night, the tours of nursing homes, and even a prison, and the fun we had along the way. Louise, Jim's wife, narrated our concerts with such sensitivity that I grew to appreciate my faith even more during these experiences." Cheryl McBride Dietrich recalled a memorable choir tour to southern California in 1970:

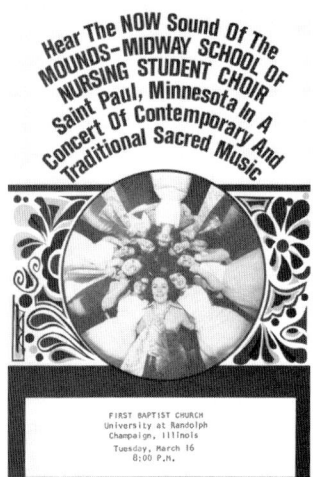

Poster for choir tour.

> We were preparing for a concert at Los Angeles Baptist. We found homeless women going through our suitcases when we returned from an afternoon in the city. That evening when we sang the song, *Lonely People*, I began to understand more about life and where the Lord calls us to live. I looked out and saw the lonely faces in the church. During this tour, we were to sing in the Watts area. The concert was canceled but we sat with four or five Black

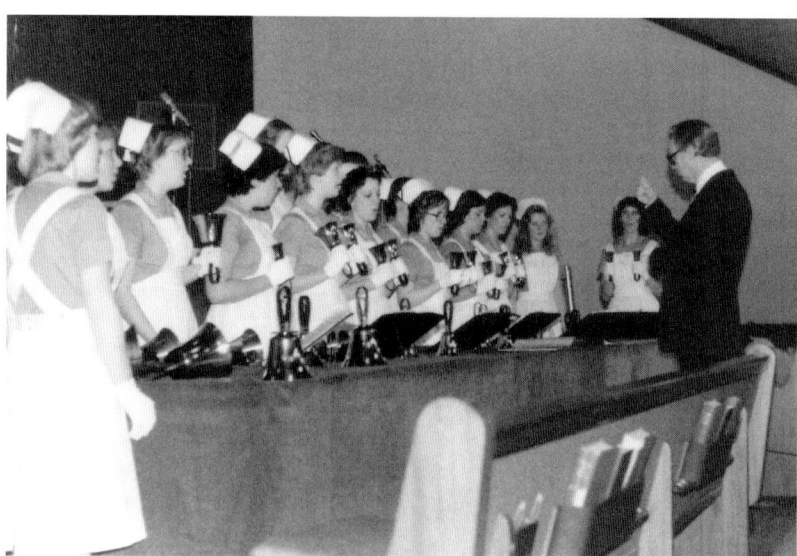

Jim Davies directs the bell ringers in 1981.

136 THIS CAP OF WHITE

Panthers who spoke about their beliefs and passions for the Watts area. We were glad to get on the bus and share with each other about what the Black Panthers had just shared. I often think of those days, I did not know what to ask when it was question time as I came from an all white community in Ohio, but it was an eye opening time for me of racial trials and problems.

In the last few years of the school, the choir took on a new name — The Healing Touch.

Spiritual life, 1970s

After Dorothy Lee left in 1971, Eunice Peterson Kronholm took over the task of counseling students. On March 15, 1974, in a terrifying series of events that made national headlines, Kronholm was kidnapped and held for ransom. After her husband received a message demanding a ransom, the Kronholm home became an FBI command post with dozens of agents listening to phone conversations and following leads. They finally made a $400,000 drop, but, as time passed and she did not appear, the family began to prepare for the worst.

All the while, Eunice had kept her composure and used her human behavior training to an advantage. She witnessed to her captors, reminding them of the difference between kidnapping and murder charges. Finally, the men released her.

Those experiences and subsequent trials became the subject for a book and a movie, *Held for Ransom*, and opened the door for Kronholm to share her testimony at clubs, churches, and civic groups throughout the Midwest. Back home, at Mounds-Midway, it gave additional meaning to her words of counsel. She wrote:

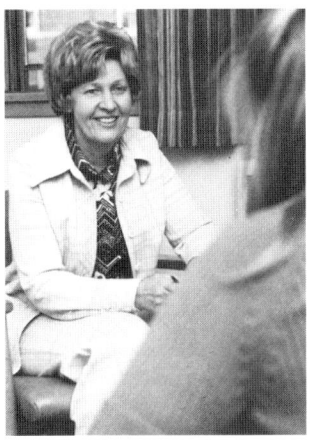

Eunice Kronholm

> Many students have come seeking help to face an exam, as if flunking that exam would be the end of the world. They are bound by their fear of a poor test grade until they can cope with a worse alternative, like a change in their vocational plans. In my experience I found this principle true. I dealt with the worst possible thing that could happen to me — death. I could only begin to cope with where I was after I was willing to say, "God, if I am to die, I'm ready."

Cheryl McBride Dietrich recalled the spiritual atmosphere that she found when she first came to Mounds-Midway. "I knew it was the right place for me," she said. "The first song that was sung by a trio of Seniors was 'Gentle Shepherd.' When I heard the words to this song at our first chapel, I knew the Lord had put me in the right place."

Faith was not without its challenges, though. Several students, years later, recalled the death of Karen Hansen in a car accident. Carol Harrison Harms said, "We were open about talking about our faith but we were not in a box." Indeed, there was a growing range of beliefs represented at the school. Stephen Trost (1975) said, "I am a Roman Catholic and as such found the Christianity I was exposed to at MMSN was very different than the faith I was raised in."

One by one, Minnesota's diploma schools closed their doors. The shuttering of St. Barnabas and St. Mary's led to the demise of the Minnesota Video Nursing Education Corporation in 1975. The state nursing board continued to press for the end of the diploma school. Following one directive in 1975, Char Olson and Mel Conley fired off a letter to its executive director, Joyce Showalter: "Diploma schools continue to receive hundreds of applicants indicating a continued interest in the programs. Since there are apparently not enough options for students, it would seem unwise to eliminate the diploma program as a choice. Of 180 of MM graduates taking these examinations in Minnesota since 1970, only one has failed to pass one part of the exam."[16]

To the public, the projected image was one of confidence, since it became more difficult to attract new students. Charlotte Olson said, "We really had to work hard, visiting schools and vocational fairs." The catalogue was compelled to remind prospective applicants that, "The American Hospital Association strongly supports hospital schools of nursing. . . . Hospital schools of nursing are truly educational in character . . . deserving recognition by the academic world and the public."

Behind the scenes, discussions continued to take place to secure a collegiate home for the nursing program. While these talks included meetings with representatives of Concordia, Macalaster, and Lakewood Colleges, the principal target remained Bethel College. In the early seventies, a planning committee initiated contact with Bethel representatives. Although initial negotiations seemed to go well, Bethel tabled the issue. As Gordon Smith reported to the Baptist Hospital Fund board, "At the present time the situation does not look good primarily because of Bethel's need for between $80,000 to $100,000 annual subsidy for the proposed program."

As a first step, however, the nursing school contracted with the college to provide science and liberal arts courses, with students receiving full academic credit. Students were bused to Bethel's new campus.[17]

Finally, with the enthusiastic support of Dean George Brushaber, the Bethel Board of Regents approved a baccalaureate nursing program in 1979. The following year, Mounds-Midway admitted its last class. Beth Peterson, who taught Fundamentals of Nursing, was one of the first faculty to leave after the class of 1981 graduated, leaving no more freshmen. She wrote, "I left to attend further school, however, for many, the closure of MMSN meant the end of their teaching careers. They were people of vision even when the cost for them personally was great."

But the enthusiasm was whole-hearted. Eleanor Edman, the first director of Bethel's nursing department, warmly recalled the reception given her by Mel Conley and Charlotte Olson. "Char Olson was just glowing that this was going to start." she recalled. "She called all the clinical facilities to introduce me and make sure that we got the Mounds-Midway place." Edman also remembered attending a retirement party for Hazel Johnson, director of the Gustavus Adolphus nursing program. "I didn't know any of the other program chairs yet. I was chatting and see this woman that I didn't know make an obvious beeline toward me. She came up to me, stuck out her hand, and said, 'I'm Wanyce Sandve. Are you the new program chair at Bethel?' I said, yes. She said, 'Praise the Lord, they finally did it!'"

Charlotte Olson, in her final report to the state nursing board, wrote:

> As you know, the closure has been considered and planned for a long time. Our faculty feels that we have had a good school and are proud of our graduates. We are very aware of the trends in health care and in nursing education and have no question about the wisdom of the decision to close the school. And yet, there is a sense of sadness as we come to the end of an era and terminate many long and good relationships.[18]

With this mixture of pride and sadness, the Mounds-Midway School of Nursing closed on May 28, 1983, following graduation ceremonies at the First Baptist Church in Saint Paul. The class motto that year read: "I shall not pass through this world but once. Any good, therefore, that

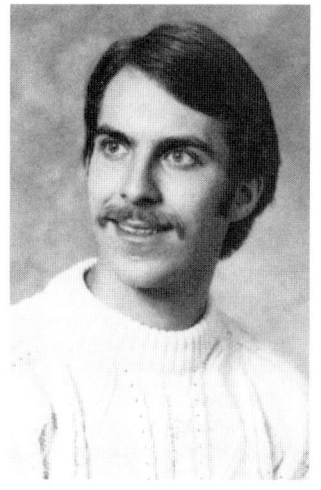

The last graduate to receive a Mounds-Midway School of Nursing diploma was Kurt Ziehlke, Class of 1983.

Chapter Four 139

I can do, or any kindness that I can show to any human being, let me do it now. Let me not defer nor neglect it, for I shall not pass this way again." Although students would no longer pass through its doors, the story of the Mounds-Midway School of Nursing is not yet over.

Endnotes

[1] Mounds-Midway News Letter 18 (May 1958), 2.
[2] "Wanyce Sandve," Obituary, *Minneapolis Star Tribune*, 5 March 2000.
[3] *Mounds-Midway School of Nursing Alumni Newsletter* (February 1997), 2.
[4] "Trustees Endorse Long Range Hospital Center Plans," *Baptist Hospital Bulletin*, 4 (May-June 1960), 1.
[5] Isabel Harris and Lettie Christenson, Report of the Survey of Mounds-Midway School of Nursing, 25-26 February 25 1959, Minnesota Board of Nursing.
[6] See Lois D. Anderson, "Use of Television in Nursing Education," *International Journal of Nursing Studies*, 7 (1970), 31-37. Also see Adella Bennett Espelien, "The Television Lecture — Then What?" *American Journal of Nursing*, 65 (1965).
[7] *Baptist Hospital Fund Bulletin*, 1962.
[8] *Annual Report, Mounds-Midway School of Nursing*, 31 December 1962. Minnesota Board of Nursing.
[9] *Educational Study Committee Report, Mounds-Midway School of Nursing. June 1965*, Minnesota Board of Nursing.
[10] James Davies, *Sing . . . with Understanding* (Chicago: Covenant Press, 1966).
[11] "Festival Thrills 52,000," *Chicago Tribune*, 19 August 1962.
[12] *Baptist Hospital Fund Bulletin*, IX (April 1965), 1-4.
[13] *Baptist Hospital Fund Bulletin*, XIV (14 June 1970), 1.
[14] L. J. Collatz, Memorandum, 18 November 1964, Minnesota Board of Nursing; Report of Ad Hoc Educational Study Committee, 31 January 1966. Bethel University Department of Nursing Archives.
[15] *The Sternum Star*, 21 May 1979.
[16] Charlotte Olson and L. Melvin Conley to Joyce Schowalter, Executive Director, Minnesota Board of Nursing, 21 March 1975.
[17] *The Final Report of the Nursing Advisory Committee: An Investigation of the Role of Education in Nursing Science at Bethel College in Cooperation with Mounds-Midway Hospitals*. February 1975. Nursing Advisory Committee, Dr. Philip Carson, chairman. Bethel University Archives.
[18] Charlotte Olson to Margaret Bach, Assistant Director, Minnesota Board of Nursing, 10 June 1983, Minnesota Board of Nursing.

CHAPTER FIVE
The Tie That Binds

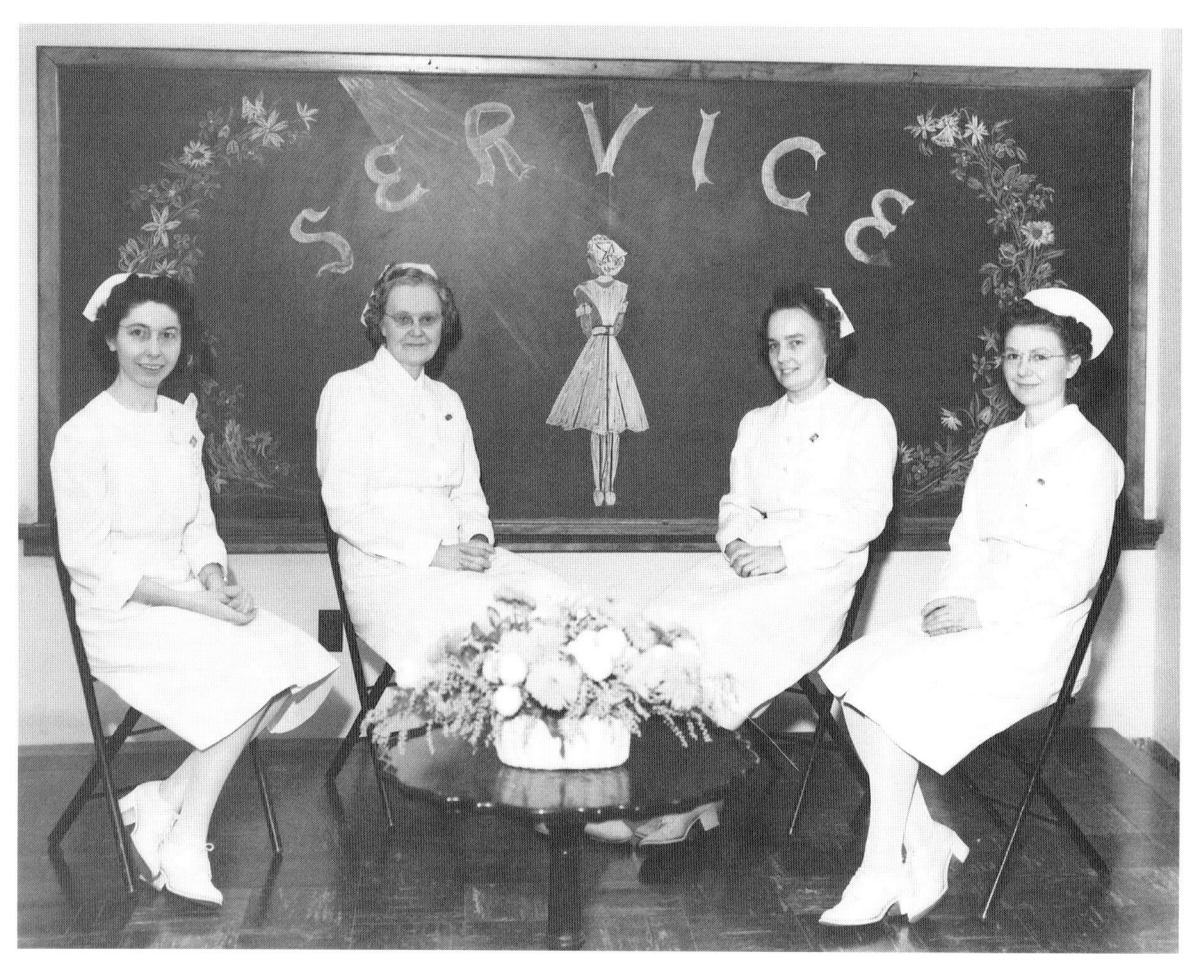

Robert Earl Hall classroom, Mounds Park. Left to right: Olivia Geidd Larson (1941), Ruth Gustafson, Violet Nelson (1936), Muriel Severson Hudek

When asked how she felt about the closing of Mounds-Midway, Adella Bennett Espelien responded, "The school might have closed, but it continues still in the lives of its graduates and in the lives of the people that they have touched." There are 2,327 stories that should be in the book, and that is just the total number of graduates. When you multiply that by the faculty and staff at the two hospitals, then include the thousands of patients and their families, you begin to understand the impact of the Mounds-Midway School of Nursing. But it also suggests how daunting the task is to tell what happened to those graduates and to assess their continuing service. A writer can only dip his hands into the deep pool of stories and pull out a few while paying honor to all.

Graduates went into nursing. On the surface, that is a simple statement, but it hardly captures the scope of work that the profession now embraces.

Look, for example, at Candyce Kuehn's career as a specialist. She graduated from Mounds-Midway School of Nursing in 1976 and then earned her bachelor's degree at Metro State University. Taking a position at the Regions Hospital Burn Center in 1976, she was a staff nurse and clinical educator prior to her promotion to nurse manager in 1982. In that position, she is responsible for day-to-day patient care, including operations, budgeting, and staffing of the inpatient and outpatient care. Well-respected in her profession and active in the American Burn Association (ABA), Candyce has authored and co-authored many scientific abstracts, moderated continuing education sessions and has been active on several ABA committees. Candyce also authored papers in the *Journal of Burn Care and Rehabilitation* and *Trauma Quarterly*. She became active in fire prevention and education, including educating first responders, emergency and inpatient personnel.

Or consider Susanne Whirley's path, which took her into community health and education away from the Twin Cities. After receiving her diploma in 1975, she pursued a bachelor's degree in nursing from Bemidji State University and later received her master's degree in advanced practice nursing from the College of St. Scholastica in Duluth with additional coursework in rural health. Whirley developed and taught community education classes in women's health, humor and healing, and neuromuscular relaxation in Wadena, then joined

Chapter Five

the Wadena Medical Center in 2006 as the clinic's family nurse practitioner.

Seventy-five years ago, a nurse typically worked in a hospital, in a physician's office, or on private duty in a home. But now the vocation reaches into all aspects of community life. Dawn Opseth Rankin (1981) became a Certified Correctional Health professional and Director of Nursing at a Medium Security Prison. Gladys George Kuehn (1957) went into nursing on the staff of Bates College in Lewiston, Maine, and later served as president of Maine College Health Association. Sandra Mudder Dean (1961) served as staff development director at Dossett Long Term Care Center in Spearfish, South Dakota, where they pioneered the first Alzheimer's care wing in an LTC facility. Janice Jackson Johnson (1953), who served on the faculty during the closing years of Mounds-Midway, later took the position as Parish Nurse at Eagle Brook Church in White Bear Lake — a new field that has attracted several graduates.

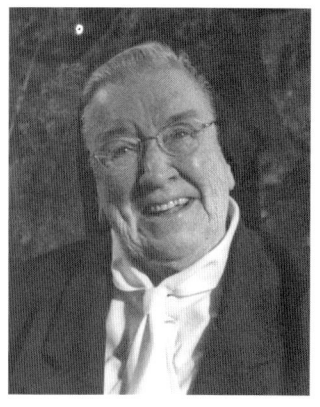

Sister Helen Kyllingstad, Class of 1938

Some graduates moved from person-to-person patient care into administration. Helen Jameson (1946), who earned bachelor's and master's degrees from the University of Minnesota, became a nurse consultant with Rochester Methodist Hospital in Rochester, Minnesota, and St. Luke's Hospital in Jacksonville, Florida, conducting operations research in nurse scheduling. Before assuming her role as nurse consultant, she was associate administrator at Rochester Methodist Hospital and head of the nursing department there.

Although she grew up in the small town of Mora, Minnesota, Irene Menassa Ericcson (1929) said that her parents wanted her to be a doctor. Instead, she embarked on a distinguished career as a nurse. As a young woman, she went to Burma as a missionary, soon placed in charge of a nursing school for native students. Returning to the United States in 1936, Irene earned a bachelor's degree from the University of Chicago, then headed to Beirut, where she took the job as surgical nursing supervisor at the American University Hospital. After fourteen years living in Damascus, she came back to work as a supervisor at George Washington Hospital in the nation's capital, rising to the post of director of nursing in 1967.[1]

One of the more interesting career paths was taken by Helen Kyllingstad (1938). After graduation, she worked in psychiatry at Mounds Park, then moved back to North Dakota to work as a public health nurse. Working in rural areas, she delivered some babies on newspapers. She recalled one baby shower where the mother-to-be excused herself to the outhouse and returned with a baby in her arms. Helen joined the sisters of Annunciation Monastery (a Benedictine order) in 1947 and served as a hospital administrator in the mining town of Beulah, North Dakota. It was located in a converted hotel with doctors scrubbing in the bathroom sink and instruments sterilized in a twenty-quart pressure cooker on the kitchen stove. In later years, she was a nurse anesthetist while serving as administrator of the Richardton Community Hospital.[2]

How good were Mounds-Midway nurses? If peer recognition is any measure, they were very, very good. Gena Testa Schottmuller (1957) received the Distinguished Service Award in 1999 from the Minnesota Association of Professionals in Infection Control. The Hawaii Nurses Association named Judy Magnuson Boomer (1962) its Maternal Child Care Nurse of the Year in 1983. Marjorie Berg (1952) was presented a similiar award by the Minnesota Nurses Association in 1982. In 2001, that organization recognized Judith Hellquist Cady (1962) with its Clinical Practice Award. Adella Espelien earned the MNA's Political Action Award for her years of work on public policy. These are only a few of the many honors bestowed on MMSN graduates.

Although students typically came from the upper Midwest, their work has taken them far afield. Pearl Jackson Myhre, a member of the class of 1918, moved down to McAllen, Texas, where she directed the local Child Clinic. She wrote, in 1948, "My patients are about 100% Latin American. Since we are only a few miles from Mexico about all I hear is Spanish." She wrote:

> At the clinic, I have over 200 patients (babies) a month. Last month, I vaccinated, inoculated, and gave typhoid booster shots to 518. The doctors donate their time. Here is our schedule: Monday, Wednesday, and Friday mornings, Sick Baby Clinics; Tuesday afternoon is a prenatal clinic with an average of 8090 patients a month; Thursday afternoons, Well Baby Clinic. The latter is my pride. I feel we are working from the right end when we try to keep them well. We have so many with dysentery, sore eyes, and malnutrition.

Alice Turk (1951) did not go as far south, landing in Perry County, Kentucky, at a hospital 140 miles southeast of Lexington and fifteen miles from any significant town. She reported back, "We do all kinds of major surgery, have a very busy OB department, a small pediatrics ward, and a nineteen-bed adult department. Every nurse does everything from dispensing medications from the pharmacy to scrubbing in surgery, watching labor patients, and doing patient care."

Agnes Weins McKenzie (1947) headed the opposite direction — north to the Cass Lake Indian Reservation, where she worked at a thirty-five bed hospital. In a letter to the the alumni newsletter, she wrote, "I've certainly been thankful for the rural nursing experience I was able to enjoy during my Senior Cadet time besides the fundamental courses at Mounds-Midway."[3]

Some worked out of the country, not as missionaries or in the military, but as civilians. Gladys Kent Clark and Esther Voetmann Brown worked in Panama following graduation in 1941. The Canal Zone played a key strategic role as the United States entered World War II. The health department, where the women worked, provided free medical care for all employees, but also assisted crewmen from the Merchant Marine — many of whom spoke neither English or Spanish. Indeed, Esther's fluency in Danish proved useful on several occasions. She recalled, "We were all subject to rotation monthly as a new schedule was posted. We received a wide range of experience in different hospitals, outpatient clinics, OB, delivery, pediatrics, EENT, surgery, etc. We operated a leper colony." With Gladys, she began a serviceman's Bible study class. Brown wrote in 1994, "From this class I met the Navy man who has now been my husband and best friend for more than half a century."

In recent years, with the advantages of air travel, MMSN nurses can rush, in an instant, to assist with medical emergencies around the globe. Following the disaster in the wake of Hurricane Katrina, Iona Stone Holsten (1957) headed with a Red Cross Disaster Action Team to a small town in Mississippi, 130 miles north of New Orleans. When she arrived, the area's homes had suffered severe damage and there was no power. Setting up a shellter at the Easthaven Baptist Church, she worked twelve-hour shifts (evening to morning) and slept when she could on the floor in the sanctuary. The evacuees, many from New Orleans, were from all ethnic backgrounds — black, white, Hispanic, oriental and Indian, rich and poor, ages three days to eighty years. Holsten said, "They arrived with acute and chronic health problems."

The local churches pitched in and six shelters were opened in Brookhaven, Mississippi. Volunteers prepared the meals, cleaned bathrooms, answered the phones and responded to the many needs of the

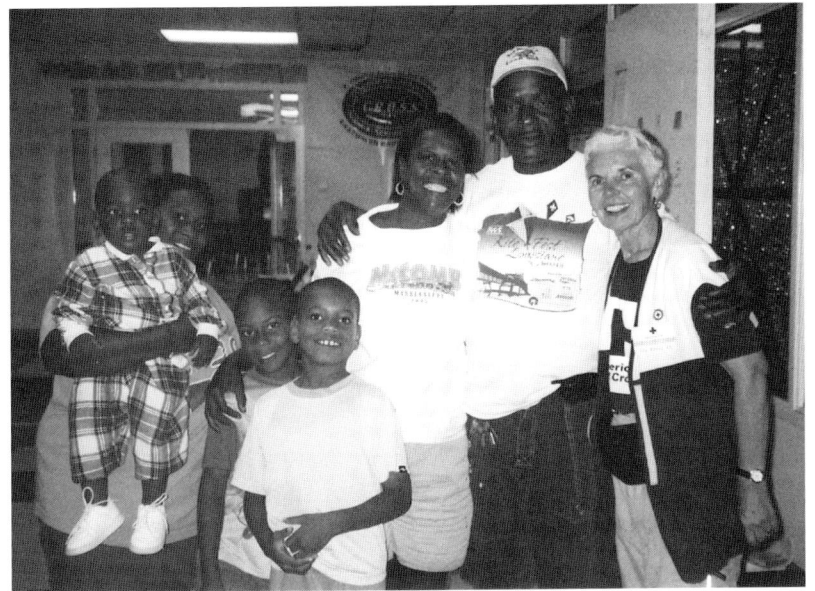

Iona Stone Holsten (1957) worked with famiilies hit by Hurricane Katrina.

evacuees. As to medical care, she wrote, "Doctors and nurses from the local hospital and from nursing homes helped us meet the health needs—URI, chronic health conditions such as diabetes, arthritis, HTN, COPD. All had to be addressed. Temperatures were taken, BP and blood sugars monitored, medications dispensed. The doctors made "house calls" to the shelters, writing prescriptions."

Other MMSN graduates have participated in similar relief operations and short-term missions. Echoing a view expressed by other Mounds-Midway graduates, Holsten said, "I enjoy making a difference in the lives of people who are hurting, comforting and giving them hope by sharing my faith."

Many alumni felt the call to teach. It was not uncommon for graduates to return to Mounds-Midway. The list is long and, hopefully, some of their stories are told in preceding chapters. Others embarked on distinguished teaching careers at other institutions.

Evelyn Ellis Cohelan (1938) headed to California after graduation. She wrote:

> When I first came to Mounds Park, I was quite shocked to find that I would have to do some psychiatric nursing before I could graduate. Deciding to take the bitter with the sweet, I stayed on. Now as I look back, that was a very wise decision for I have certainly used that experience. California has been very slow in requiring

Chapter Five 147

psychiatric experience in the basic curriculum for student nurses. As a result I found I had a skill that many California nurses did not have.

Working in the psychiatric ward in the general hospital (Herrick Memorial) in Berkeley, she determined that the field had been changing rapidly and decided to return for further education.

> I discovered many things had happened in psychiatry since 1938 so decided to see if I could catch up by going to school. With the aid and encouragement of my husband, I got my B.S. degree from the University of California in 1951. I then did a year of field work at Langley Porter Clinic on the Medical Campus of the University of California. In the fall of 1952 I began on my M.S. degree and finished in June 1953. My work has all been done in nursing education with emphasis on teaching psychiatric nursing. As part of the work for the M.S. degree I developed a teaching program in psychosomatic nursing for student nurses in the University of California School of Nursing in San Francisco.

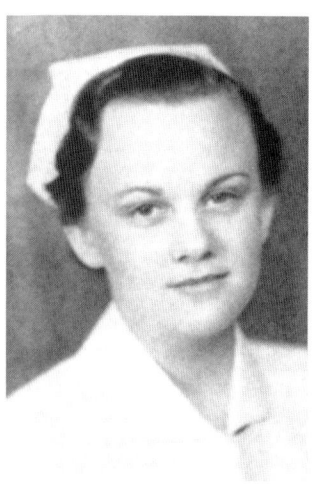

Evelyn Ellis Cohelan, Class of 1938

Cohelan had bigger things in store. Her husband, Jerry, was elected to Congress in 1958 — a position he held for twelve years — and the family moved to the Washington, D.C. area. To some, being a congressman's wife could be a heady prospect — one that could consume much of her time — but she still wanted to be a nurse, to learn, and to teach. She said, "I tried it — the daily luncheons, teas, receptions. And I tried League of Women Voters and the PTA. They're fine for some people but I wanted an area where I felt I could do more." She took a position at the University of Maryland, becoming dean of that prominent nursing program's graduate school, while earning her Ph.D. from Berkeley in 1963. In the 1970s, a call came to organize a school of nursing at George Mason University in Fairfax, Virginia. Few have the opportunity to start a program from scratch, but she jumped at the chance, heading the nursing school for eight years until her retirement in 1981. She has been called "one of the grand dames of nursing education."

Two graduates, Lois D. Anderson (1946) and Dagmar Swanburg Brodt (1941), received what might be the highest honor to be given a nurse: election to the American Academy of Nursing. The AAN is comprised of 1,500 nurse leaders who are literally at the top of their

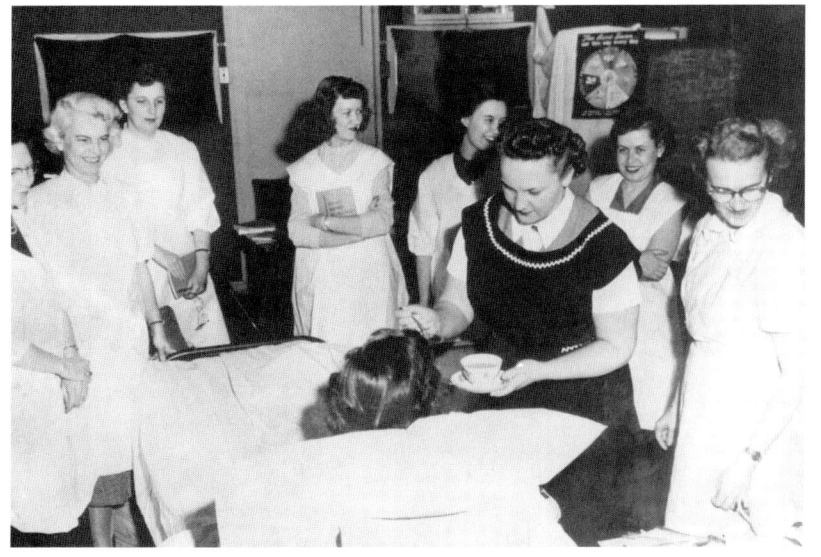

Dagmar Brodt (1941) instructs Red Cross volunteers in Matsushima, Japan in 1953.

profession, having accomplished extraordinary milestones in their nursing careers. AAN members are elected by their peers to be the best and the brightest in the nursing discipline.

After graduating from Mounds-Midway, Dagmar Brodt continued to work as a nurse, all the while pursuing further education and assisting her husband's work with the Red Cross. In 1945, she earned a B.S. from the University of Minnesota, followed by a M.S.N. and Ph.D. from Saint Louis University in 1963. She held teaching positions at schools as diverse as Howard University and the Medical College of Georgia. At Livingston University, she established a new school of nursing in 1973. Widely-respected for her thoughtful and incisive analysis of the nursing profession, she worked for many years at the Nursing Research Department, Naval Medical Research Institute, Bethesda, Maryland. She also authored a standard textbook, *Medical-Surgical Nursing and the Nursing Process* (Boston: Little Brown, and Company, 1986).

Other doctorates include Edna Esther Johnson (1958), who earned a Ph.D. from University of South Carolina, and taught community health in the Nurse Practitioner Program at the University of Connecticut for twenty-eight years.

As nursing entered the late twentieth century, medicine began to better understand and accept the spiritual dimensions of healing—something taught in practice at Mounds Park and Midway Hospitals. Eleanore Anderson Vogel (1950) worked with early study groups when this category of "alterations in faith" (and later called spiritual distress) was proposed and adopted. Soon after, the American

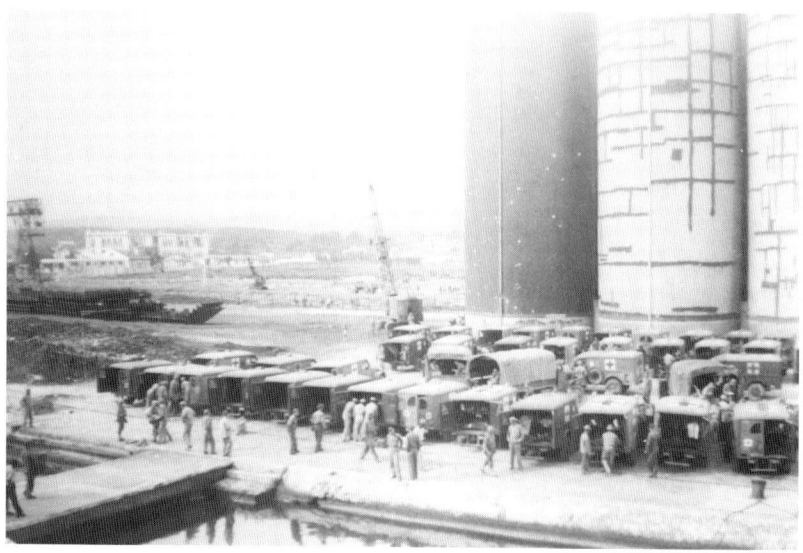

Ambulances at the docks in Bizerte, North Africa, waiting for the Shamrock to unload casuaties from Italy.

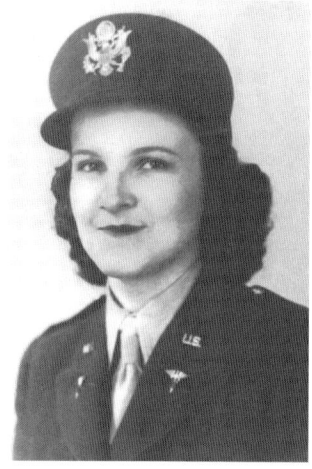

Helene Stewart Robertson

Journal of Nursing published a landmark monograph that gave professional recognition to the field as a legitimate subject for study.

Marilyne Backlund Gustafson (1954), with a doctorate from Walden University, helped to bring the role of spiritual care into the mainstream of nursing education through her teaching and writing. Gustafson, who taught at the University of Minnesota School of Nursing for three decades, introduced spiritual care into that school's curriculum — a key step in breaking the subject out into secular education. In addition, she contributed to the field in several Nurses Christian Fellowship publications and at seminars to teach spiritual care here and at international conferences. Elizabeth Peterson (1971), on the faculty at Bethel University's School of Nursing, has also written on spiritual needs in psychiatric nursing and the elderly.[4]

Military Service

Mounds-Midway nurses answered the call to serve when the nation went to war, beginning with World War I.

During World War II, dozens of the school's graduates worked on battlefields in the European, Mediterranean, and Pacific theaters, with some helping in Japanese and European relocation camps, while others served in mainland military hospitals.

Stationed aboard the hospital ship *Shamrock*, Helene Stewart Robertson (1942) sailed to the Mediterranean in September 1943, shortly after the initial Allied invasion of Italy. As they approached the coast near Salerno, she wrote in her diary, "We are now only fifteen miles from where the heavy fighting is going on. . . . So far, we have no patients but with the fighting so near, I think we will get a lot of fresh casualties."

The casualties came, and the *Shamrock* loaded the wounded soldiers up and ferried them to hospitals behind the lines in Sicily and North Africa. "About two hundred ambulances came down from one of the hospitals and [in] only two and one-half hours, all our patients were unloaded," Helene wrote. "I feel extremely sorry for these boys and all boys that have to suffer, and their families, as a result of man's unadulterated insanity, war."

The back and forth trips continued and over the next six months, the *Shamrock* evacuated 12,263 soldiers. Sometimes they found themselves in harm's way.

> At 7 p.m. we took ringside seats in hell! Six waves of German planes attacked Naples while we sat here in the harbor. The flares were dropped and the 90mm anti-aircraft immediately opened up. The sky became a fireworks display and bombs were dropping all around. The tracer bullets blazed long trails up into the heavens and we saw two German planes shot down. Shrapnel was flying wildly and landed on our decks. . . . My reaction was not one of fear — nor was any of the nurses', but rather a strange feeling of excitement and wonder.

Helene Stewart Robertson served until the end of the war, marrying fellow crew member Edward Robinson in October 1944. For her service, she was awarded a campaign medal for the Mediterranean theater as well as the Bronze Star.

In that same month, Margaret Edwards Radmann (1938) was with the Allied invasion forces in northern France and Belgium. Then came the German counterattack, later known as the Battle of the Bulge. "The big push came and we were really in it," she wrote in a letter home. "In less than twelve hours the whole division moved and we six nurses came right along in. [I] will never forget that long drive through the night with no lights, up and down those mountain roads, knowing the Jerries were closing in pretty fast."

She told her friends, "[I] will never forget this Christmas. Christmas eve we were told that we were only one and one-half miles from the fighting. . . . Right now we have only one surgery set up for emergency amputations and such. Two nurses work on post-operative wards, one

Chapter Five 151

on night duty, and I work in shock. When the patients come in, they get blood, plasma, and oxygen. We cut off their wet clothes and roll them in warm, dry blankets."

By late winter 1945, the crisis passed, Edwards noted the rain melting the deep snows, uncovering "bodies of our dead Americans, Jerries, cows and horses. It is all very sickening." For solace, she turned to her old friends from Mounds-Midway. "I am always glad when the newsletter comes," she wrote. "One of the best morale builders there is."[5]

Meanwhile, in the Pacific, Allied forces continued to move closer, island by island, to the Japanese mainland. The hospitals were typically removed from the immediate fighting and located on islands in the rear. That is where Violet Isaacson Swackhammer (1941) found herself in early 1945. Stationed on the Mariana Islands, she worked in a medical war "with mostly chronic arthritis and such." Enjoying "my nice South Pacific sunshine" she reveled that "there is always something to do and plenty of places to deposit a group of girls for an evening." To her Mounds-Midway friends she reported, "The Sunday services out on deck were really an inspiration. Quite unlike a real one though with shirt sleeves rolled up, bare and brown topped boys, and perspiration running down everyone." However, the battles for the islands of Iwo Jima and Okinawa followed and casualties began to fill the wards.[6]

Myrtle Nereson Quamen (1939) was a veteran of some of the bitterest fighting in World War II. When her training at Mounds-Midway was finished, she took a position as an office nurse in Sacramento, California. With the war, that city became a major depot center for troops, creating a demand for nurses. She enlisted and, following training, was sent overseas, arriving in Africa on March 27, 1944. Assigned to an Evacuation Hospital with the 5th Army, she came into contact for the first time with American soldiers wounded in battle. In a few months, Lt. Nereson was transferred to Italy, this time to a General Hospital about thirty miles behind the front lines. Lt. Nereson received a Battle Star for the Rome-Arno campaign.

Nereson then became part of the rear units of the invasion forces in France. Moving into France on D-Day plus 9 she joined the 51st Evacuation Hospital with the 7th Army, located only five or six miles behind the front lines in one of three "leap frog" evacuation hospitals. These hospitals, set up in tents, were spaced so that when the front moved forward the last "evac" hospital jumped the two forward ones to a position just rear of the fighting, the process was repeated as the Medical Corps followed the line of battle.

Like Margaret Edwards, Nereson was also near the front lines during the Battle of the Bulge. When other hospital units were pulled back, she remained with fifty other nurses to care for patients in a one thousand-bed hospital. The Germans bombed and strafed but the hospital continued to give medical aid, working under "blackout" conditions and improvising countless necessities. As one of five nurse supervisors, Lt. Nereson received the Bronze Star for meritorious service during this period.

When Germany fell in May of 1945, Lt. Nereson remained in the occupied country for six more months. She was promoted to Captain in this theater. For her service during World War II, Capt. Nereson holds, in addition to the Bronze Star, battle stars for Rome-Arno, Southern France, the Rhineland, and Central Europe.

Although it appears that no Mounds-Midway graduates served in Korea during that conflict, Nereson had an impact on its medical service. She was assigned to that country shortly after World War II. As Chief Nurse at the 382nd Station Hospital located between Inchon and Seoul, she began to train Korean women to become military nurses. Under her leadership, and working with an interpreter, she trained two classes to become qualified nurses, often relying on example. Although Korean nurses had never been recognized by the International Nurses Association, eight of Nereson's students passed their examinations and became 2nd Lieutenants in the Korean Army Nurse Corps. She remained in Korea for two years. Reminiscing on her years of service, she said, "I think it was then I realized that if I had to choose over again, I'd still be a nurse for Uncle Sam."

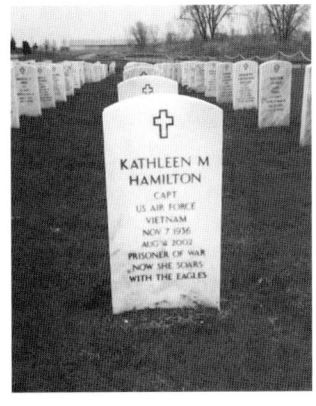

Kathleen McNaughton Hamilton's grave at Fort Snelling.

More than 6,200 women served as Army nurses in Vietnam. Often unsung heroines, they worked on military installations and sometimes in remote hospitals. Among them was Kathleen McNaughton Hamilton (1957), who saw two wars, one as a child and one as a military nurse. Her parents were Christian and Missionary Alliance missionaries, assigned to what was then known as French Indochina. As the Japanese moved through southeast Asia, the family, now with three small children, sought refuge in the Philippines. But it proved only a momentary respite.

After attempting to hide when the Japanese took over the country, Kathleen's father ultimately surrendered, along with his family. There were shipped to a Prisoner of War camp near Manila, where they remained until the arrival of American forces in February 1945. "She was quite traumatized," her sister said about those years.

When U.S. involvement in Vietnam expanded from the assignment of a few advisors to a full-blown war, Hamilton joined the Air Force in 1965, eager to serve because she was "really grateful to the soldiers who rescued her in the Philippines." Stationed at the massive Cam Rahn Bay military base, she was relatively safe throughout her year in Vietnam, but was in the country during the 1968 Tet Offensive.

After Vietnam, Hamilton used the G.I. Bill to get a degree in psychology at the University of Minnesota. She worked after that with chemical dependency at Abbott Northwestern Hospital in Minneapolis, and later with Ebenezer Health care homes in Minneapolis before her death.[7]

Valerie Buchan (1957) retired as a Colonel and received the Bronze Star. She recalled that in 1964, "I saw an article in Look or Life magazine with three flag-draped coffins and read about these advisors who had been killed. I asked my family, "Where is Vietnam?" As American involvement escalated over the next year, she decided to go and serve.

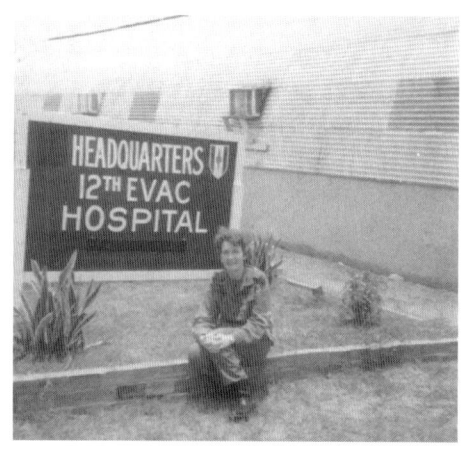

Valerie Buchan (1957) in Vietnam.

I contacted all three branches. The Air Force stalled and hemmed and hawed about whether they would accept me, but the Army called right away and said we'd like to send a staff car over for you. They did and brought me to their office and explained the service to me. When I returned home, I got a call from the Air Force, saying that they were ready to go ahead. I said that I had pretty much made up my mind to go with the Army. A little while later, the doorbell rang and here were two Air Force men in uniform, including a pilot who looked a lot like Rock Hudson.

Although an effective recruiting technique for some, it left Valerie undeterred and she joined the Army.

After two years in Japan, caring for many war casualties, she volunteered to go to Vietnam. She was assigned to a base west of Saigon and just above the Mekong Delta. She recalled, "Base camp was like a small town with the hospital in the middle. We lived in wood 'hooches' and worked twelve-hour shifts. There was no place to go and we shared everything. I missed that [camaraderie and closeness] when I got home."

As support for 25th Infantry Division, the base hospital cared for wounded flown by helicopter directly from the battlefield to the hospital. Buchan said, "Our job was mainly to stabilize them in the emergency room. It was the biggest challenge of my nursing career."

There were also emotional and moral issues. She recalled one case, "Soon after I got there, they brought in a young kid from Illinois and we just worked on him and worked on him but we couldn't save him. I picked up his ID card and it was his twenty-first birthday. I almost lost it and decided that I wouldn't look at them anymore." On the base, they also treated some civilians — women and children — as well as a few prisoners-of-war. Buchan thought about the dilemma of giving aid to an enemy. "Morally, you do what they need but the attitude is completely different."

She reflected on her education, saying, "I became thankful for my training at MMSN. We learned how to handle things and we had good organizational skills."

Another Mounds-Midway graduate, Betty Stahl Doebbeling (1962), served in Vietnam as both as civilian and as soldier. Volunteering for the USAID, she remembered, "I was excited. I wasn't far from thirty and I hadn't traveled yet in life. I hadn't seen the Twin Cities until after high school. I'd be the first in the family to travel anywhere."

That wish was soon fulfilled because, after a crash immersion course in the language, she flew to Saigon in June 1967. She was assigned to the Can Tho Provincial Hospital, where she lived and worked for the next eighteen months, first in ortho, then in a burn ward. Her main duty was to nurse the civilian population back to health. She sometimes traveled into the surrounding countryside, bringing basic medical care and medicine to local villages.

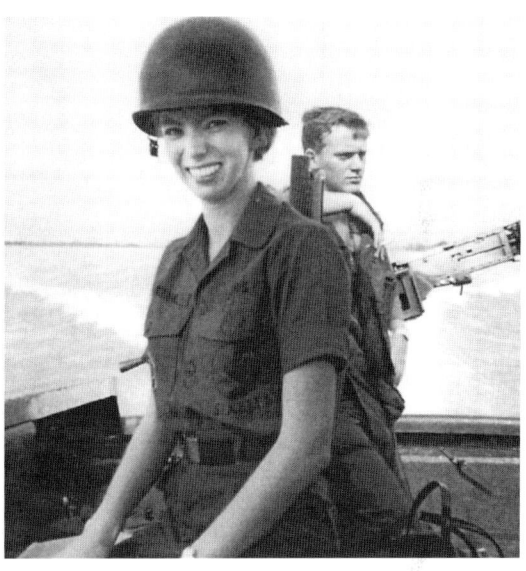

Betty Stahl Doebbeling on the Mekong Delta, 1967.

The war came to her doorstep during the Tet offensive in early 1968. Fearing for their lives, the nurses remained in their apartment building while fighting went on all around them. "We really didn't think we'd survive," she recalled. "There was no way for us to escape. I wrote a letter to my parents, telling them we had no weapons and no guards." During the tense days that followed, the women rationed their food and kept watch.

Finally, the Viet Cong pulled back, but she was never far from danger.

Chapter Five 155

"We'd hear gunfire and rockets all the time, at least four or five nights a week," she said. "And you'd always wonder if this one was coming to get you. I would lay on the floor and hide under my mattress. It was hard to live with the thought that you might die the next day."

Near the end of her eighteen-month tour with USAID, Doebbeling visited a military hospital and decided to join the Army. After basic training, she was assigned to the 312th Evac in Chu Lai, north of Saigon, where she served for a one-year tour of duty. She left the country with the rank of captain and later received a Bronze Star for her meritorious service.

Looking back on her Vietnam experiences, she said, "It made me grow up. You really become an adult going through all of that and see a different side of humanity. It taught me what's really important in life and to cope when you have next to nothing."[8]

Captain Kurt Ziehlke (1983) continued Mounds-Midway's record of service into the most recent American conflict in Iraq. Kurt was in charge of the Post Anesthesia Care Unit with the 915th Forward Surgical Team—a front-line unit stabilizing wounded soldiers. Besides his medical care for the soldiers, he assisted Iraqi civilians

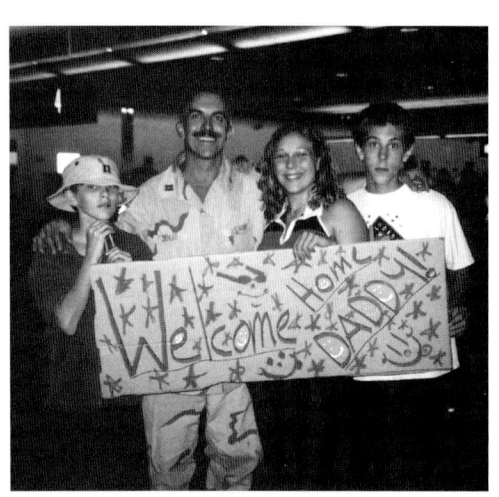

Kurt Ziehlke (1983) was greeted by his family when he returned from duty in Iraq.

and prisoners of war. "One Iraqi soldier had his hands bound and was scared," Ziehlke said. "I read to him from a phrase book to let him know that he was a POW and that he would be treated well. We wound up exchanging pictures of our enemies but there was no reason to hate each other."

On the evening of July 3, 2004, after heading to bed, he heard several explosions nearby when a shell hit some camouflage netting hung over the sleeping area. Ziehlke had jumped from his cot after the second round and was about to dive under the nearest Humvee when the third hit. Ziehlke was thrown through the air onto the bumper of a Humvee, wrenching his back and knocking him unconscious. In spite of a back injury and a shrapnel wound to his shoulder, Ziehlke was able to give emergency first aid to the others. Although the chair he had just left was blown-up and the blanket and mosquito netting over his bed were in shreds, he had moved in the nick of time. "The next morning," he recalled, "when I looked around at the Humvees, the tent, my computer . . . there were holes everywhere, even shrapnel in my blanket."[9]

His unit returned home shortly after the incident and Ziehlke was awarded the Purple Heart.

Missionaries

The school had a long, consistent commitment to missions, sending out eighty-three career missionaries. They represent more than thirty-two boards, serving in some fifty-seven countries plus the United States. The length of service ranged from one to more than fifty years.

Few missionaries were more beloved than Laura Reddig, a 1934 Mounds-Midway graduate. Born in North Dakota in 1912, she graduated from Mounds-Midway and had additional education at the Baptist Missionary Training School in Chicago. Following graduation in June 1938, convinced that she was called to Cameroon, she told the denominational general secretary, who promptly tried to discourage her. A BMTS teacher, Alethea Kose, spelled out the obstacles, telling her, "Laura, if you insist on going . . . you may be cutting your life short." Kose later remembered Reddig standing up straight and declaring, "Even if I die the day after I arrive, I still know God has called me to that field." With that response, the North American Baptist Conference sent her to Cameroon where she served for forty years.

As a missionary nurse, Reddig was involved as a teacher and a midwife. With travel restricted because of World War II, in her early years, she served with only one other couple. A friend recalled, "During those years, your letters included such things as 'Today I helped to build a bridge,' or 'Today I supervised the building of a school,' or 'Today I performed surgery.'" In 1951, she opened the first leprosy treatment center in the village of New Hope. For her work, she received the British Medal of Honor, conferred on her by Queen

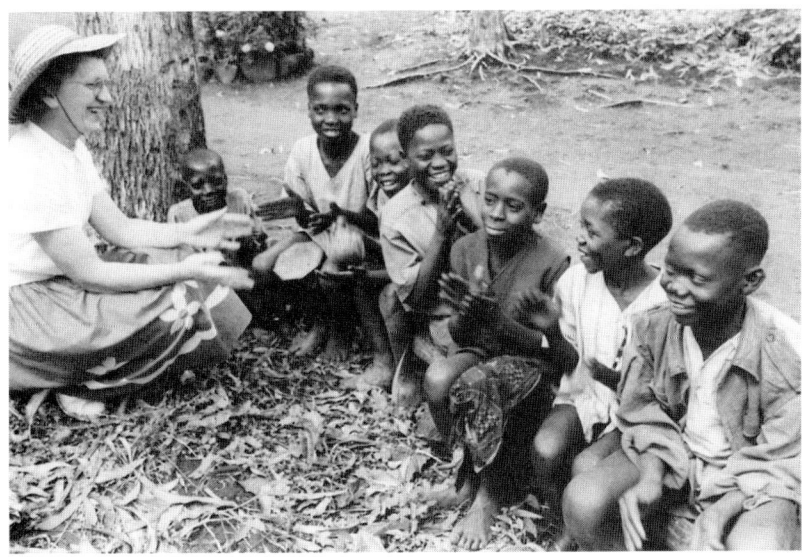

Laura Reddig, missionary to Cameroon

Elizabeth, the Cameroon Medal of Merit from the President of the United Republic of Cameroon, and the Doctor of Humanities degree from North American Baptist Seminary in Sioux Falls, South Dakota.

On a trip to Cameroon, West Africa, in early 2007, a young pastor wrote back to his church about his visit to the little village of New Hope. "Every time I visit New Hope," he told them, I am humbled, shaken, angry, and fall in love with Jesus all over again. There are not many people left at New Hope, but those that are taught us some great lessons."

Influenced by Laura Reddig's work, Barbara Kieper (1953) also served as a missionary in Cameroon after learning midwifery at the Frontier Nursing Service in rural Kentucky. She described how she put that training to use:

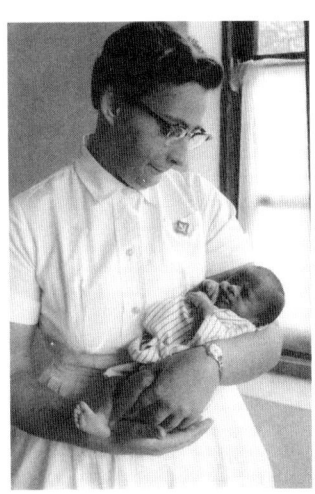

Barbara Kieper (1953) holds a premature baby after a bath at Baptist Hospital, Cameroon, in 1961.

> I was called one night to a kitchen for a woman in labor. They had a fire going giving some light but it was really smoky and the globe of the kerosene lamp was black with soot. (I forgot to bring a battery lamp.) After we moved her from the floor to a bed, I heard a lot of rustling in the walls and turned my lamp to see the walls crawling with cockroaches. Soon after that the patient delivered. I also did a delivery in a cornfield. Eventually the people built a dispensary maternity center that was very nice.

Later, when the government took over the hospital, she helped to start a health care program with an emphasis on prenatal care and immunizations.

Missionary work means much more than simply sending Americans into foreign countries. A native of the Democratic Republic of Congo (Zaire), Yema Museu Luhahi (1972) came to Mounds-Midway for her nursing diploma. After her time in Saint Paul, she earned a B.S. from St. Francis College in Joliet, Illinois, and then a master degree in Public Health from Benedictine University in Lisle, Illinois. Returning to her homeland, Yema was a lecturer, and at one time, Director of the Nursing Program at the government Higher Institute of Allied Health Sciences in Kinshasa. She served eight years (1984-1992) as a director of the General Board of Global Ministries from the Central Conference. Four of those eight years she served as a director of Women's Division.

The Luhahis became missionaries in 1992 when the United Methodist Church assigned them to Kenya as International Persons in Mission. In that capacity Yema taught at the Maua Methodist Hospital Nursing

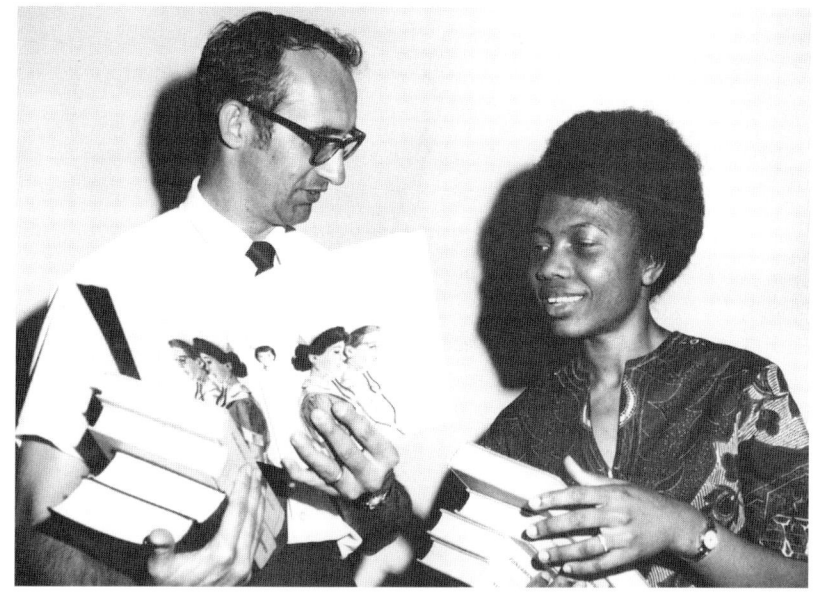

Yema Museu Luhahi, 1972, with Dr. James Fett. Fett was missionary to Congo.

School. In 1993 the Luhahis were appointed Missionary Interpreters in Residence throughout the USA for five years prior to going back to the mission field in Kenya. In 1999 Yema moved to the Maua Methodist Hospital Nursing School as a full time teaching staff, also teaching some health related courses at the Kenya Methodist University (KEMU) in Meru. Her work included organizing workshops and seminars covering subjects such as alcohol and drug abuse, education and awareness on HIV/AIDS, and the empowerment (social and economic) of women. Kenya Methodist University asked her to establish and then manage a university health clinic. When it opened its doors in 1999, the clinic had only one part-time nurse. By 2005, the university clinic, renamed University Health Center, had grown to include a well-equipped laboratory and six full time staff members.

"As I train the nurses to serve the community," said Luhahi, "we are bringing the warm and the healing light of God's love to people through our ministry of caring. By obeying Jesus' call to do unto 'the least of these.'" She concluded, "I believe that God's mission is being carried out as Jesus' love flows through our healing ministry to touch people."

When we read letters from Mounds-Midway missionaries, describing their work more than fifty years ago, we sometimes gain an insight into issues as fresh as the morning newspaper. Elaine Berdan Carpenter (1948) served in Nigeria and Dahomey with the Sudan Interior Mission. In a letter back to Mounds-Midway, she wrote:

Chapter Five

> I believe that it would please God to break down this awful barrier of Mohammedanism, even as He broke down the walls of mighty Jericho. I am sure that it will cost all of us something. It will cost us time in prayer, wrestling with God for the souls of men. The medical work is such a help in winning the confidence of these people. How we praise Him for this opening. But we come to the end of ourselves as we realize that only the Spirit of God can break through to a soul and bring it to Christ.

With her husband, Charles, she continued to do evangelistic work while running a dispensary among the Fulani people.

There has been a special bond between Mounds-Midway School of Nursing and Tezpur, India, since the Baptist Christian Hospital opened as a dispensary in 1952, growing to a thirty-six bed facility within two years. In that year, two MMSN graduates, Arlene Jensen Callaway (1943) and Betty Person (1950) founded a School of Nursing, soon joined by Ruby Eliason (1951), then followed two years later by Ruth Bertell (1953).

For the next twenty-five years, Ruby Eliason served at the Baptist Christian Hospital. Under her leadership, the school gained the respect of the local community and the Indian government. Her friend and associate, Elsa Knudsen, explained that there was more to the school than just a technical education: "The witness of the hospital was the most important reason for its existence."

But it was not always easy and Eliason was no plaster saint. "When I went home on my first furlough," she wrote, "I was empty, bitter, and absolutely fatigued. I had gone to India thinking missionaries were super-spiritual people, not human beings. God used the time back... to straighten me out."[10]

Eliason held high standards for the school and pressed ahead with her own education. During furloughs, she completed her B. S. N. in 1961 and her Master's in Nursing at the University of Washington in 1968. Knudsen talked about her leadership, saying, "I would like to emphasize Ruby's leadership in the hospital, school of nursing and Bible Study among students and staff. Only eternity will reveal the results of her dedicated work in these areas — especially her leadership in the spiritual lives of all of us."

Turning the leadership over to a national nurse, Eliason stepped down in 1979. Ruby's story, though, was not done. Upon leaving India

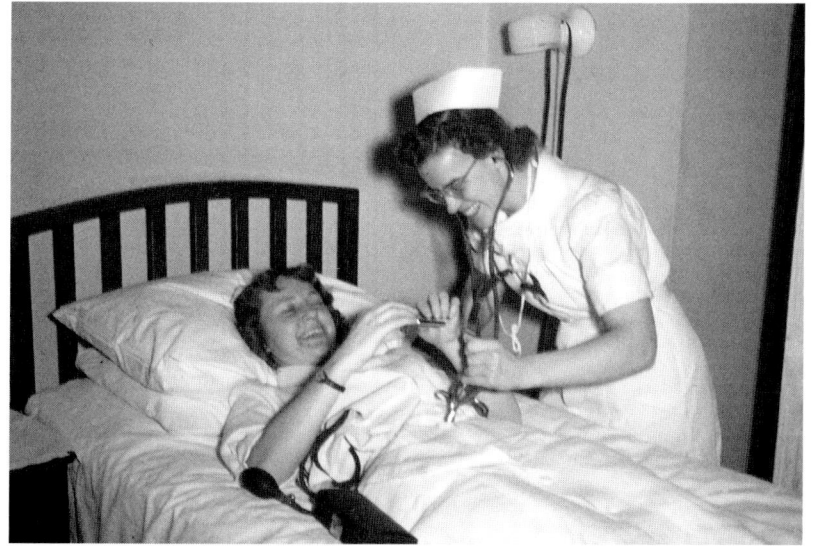

Two future missionaries, Elaine Westlund Coleman (1950) and Ruby Eliason (1951), enjoy a light-hearted moment while working at Mounds Park Hospital in 1952.

in 1980, Ruby continued to further her education, completing a M.A. in Public Health at Loma Linda University in 1982 and a Ph.D. from William Carey International University in 1996. This was not an idle academic pursuit. She continued missionary work, this time as an educational advisor with the Life Abundant Program in Cameroon. LAP was a church-related primary health care organization, sponsored by that country's Baptist Convention Health Board. Its methodology, developed with her help, encouraged community self-reliance and decision-making.

She and Dr. Laura Edwards, her longtime friend and associate, were visiting Cameroon when they were both killed in a car accident in April 2000. John Piper, in his book, *Don't Waste Your Life*, told of the lesson that he learned from this moment:

> Ruby was over eighty. Single all her life, she poured it out for one great thing: to make Jesus Christ known among the unreached, the poor, and the sick. Laura was a widow, a medical doctor, pushing eighty years old, and serving at Ruby's side in Cameroon. The brakes failed, the car went over a cliff, and they were both killed instantly. Was that a tragedy? Two lives, driven by one great passion, namely, to be spent in unheralded service to the perishing poor for the glory of Jesus Christ — even two decades after most of their American counterparts had retired to throw away their lives on trifles. No. That is not a tragedy. These lives were not wasted.

Chapter Five

And these lives were not lost. "Whoever loses his life for my sake and the Gospel's will save it" (Mark 8:35).[11]

The Tezpur hospital and school still continue their work more than fifty years after their humble beginning, but still with the support from the MMSN Alumni Association.

Mounds-Midway graduates served in other parts of Asia as well. For example, Marjorie Siemens Geary (1955) taught Indonesian nursing students. In the work, her thoughts often returned to her old school of nursing. She wrote, "As I began to teach [them] to give baths, back rubs and make tight beds with a toe pleat, I thought of Miss Violet Nelson. As I translated parts of a medical surgical nursing textbook from English into Indonesian, I remembered my teachers. As I demonstrated and supervised loving patient care, Miss Hemmes came to mind. Soap at every sink was expected, an unheard of practice in Indonesia as soap was too precious to be left just "sitting around." In addition to teaching, she worked in village health and evangelism with her husband, Wendell, a medical doctor.

For eleven years, Beverly Fillips Donner (1953), along with her husband, Fred, worked for Wycliffe Bible Translators in Vietnam. She remembered,

> There were days during my time as the anesthetist on a Public Health Service Surgical Team caring for civilian casualties in Vietnam when truck loads of people would arrive and as they were unloaded we saw what war did to the human body. Our operating room in the local hospital was primitive, had no air conditioning and our general surgeons did the orthopedic, thoracic and even neurosurgery because that's what was needed. Once again I was often administering ether because it was the only inhalation agent readily available, and for monitoring, a BP cuff and stethoscope.

They left the country only when American forces completely withdrew in April 1975.

On this side of the Atlantic, Ruth Huber Baxter (1954) worked at Hospital Vozandes, in Quito, Equador, for forty years. Ruth credited another MMSN missionary with the inspiration to enter the mission field. She wrote, "Ruby Eliason was one tremendous supervisor. She encouraged me in my spiritual walk and followed me at the end of my senior year and was instrumental in getting me to attend Moody Bible Institute. Her encouragement to fulfill my calling into missionary service and emphasizing the importance of preparation was fundamental to me and is the core of my happiest days in serving Him in Quito, Ecuador with Radio Station HCJB."

When Baxter arrived on the field in November 1964, she was placed in charge of the OR, Delivery Room Suite, Sterilization and Recovery. This heavy responsibility was complicated by the fact that she was still learning Spanish, adjusting to a new culture, and, at the time, was four months pregnant. Describing the work, she noted,

> One minute I was instrumenting for a general surgery case, then I would have to switch to orthopedics and then go to a delivery, or ENT or ear surgery. I kept thinking how I wished I could have had more training in every area. How grateful I was for the five weeks I gained in my senior year at Mounds-Midway in Surgery.

Later, as the quality of medical services improved, she became part of an operative team, with a twenty-four-hour staff and anesthesiologists on call. Still, on any given day, they might have handled hip replacements, cardiology, ENT, and gynecological procedures. Baxter retired in 2003.

Missions' work has not been limited to foreign countries. One graduate, Gwendolyn Ticknor (1934), made a big impact in a small place. With her friend and fellow nurse, Minnie Scott, she moved to rural Arkansas as "faith" missionaries, living a simple life and ministering to their neighbors, both physically and spiritually. A 1946 Arkansas Gazette article called the pair, "carpenters, farm women and odd-jobbers by will power, necessity, and the grace of God."

They built their own home, using an old 1935 Chevrolet plus a team of horses and a wagon, they hauled nineteen loads of rock for the foundation, put up the walls and roof, did all the wiring, and built the chimney and fireplace. To provide good drinking water, they dug a hole and built their own cistern. They also constructed a cow and goat shed, a garage, and other outbuildings. To support themselves, they planted a vegetable garden and an orchard and raised goats, a cow, and a few pigs.

As nurses, they provided basic care to the neighboring families, administering shots against typhoid, diphtheria, and whooping cough

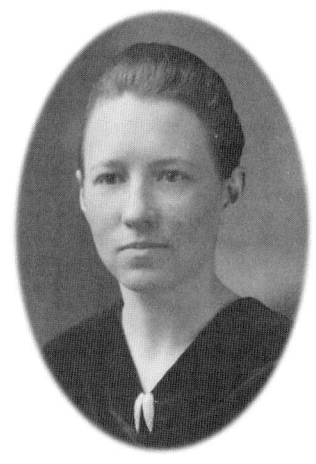

Gwendolyn Ticknor (1934) worked as a "faith missionary" in Arkansas for twenty-one years.

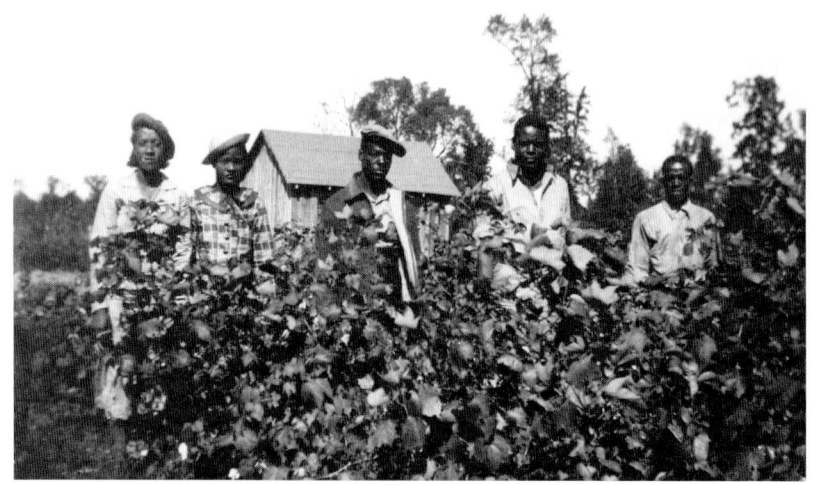

Right: A photograph taken by Ticknor while in missions' work in rural Arkansas.

every two years. As midwives, they attended more than a hundred obstetrical cases. In their home they held clinics for babies and children of pre-school age. They also taught classes in care of the sick as well as the standard Red Cross course.

As missionaries, they traveled from town to town during the summer, conducting week-long Vacation Bible Schools, combining Bible lessons with instruction in woodworking and sewing. In their spare time, they organized two church congregations. The work left local observers in awe. A reporter for the *Arkansas Gazette* wrote:

> To Miss Scott and Miss Ticknor, living modestly at Union Hill, it is the best way to achieve their aim, a life of service. They covet no fortune, they expect no praise for what they do, sincerely believing that theirs is the Lord's work, and that if they ask in faith, He will grant them strength to carry on. For along with all the many hard tasks and hours of service to the community, they have found there unlimited opportunities for friendship — and lasting associations which far more than repay their efforts.[12]

She continued her work in Union Hill for twenty-one years.

Mounds-Midway graduates have not limited their service to the field of nursing.

A Mounds-Midway education led to a career as an attorney for Sandra Barton Brisley (1982). A graduate of the William Mitchell School of Law, she worked at the University of Minnesota hospital in pediatrics and intensive care before becoming a lawyer. With that combination of skills, she gained a position at United Health Care in litigation management.

After working as a nurse, Kathryn Linn Dadukian (1964) obtained a B.A. in Finance from Marymount-Manhattan College and began a new career. As an actuarial assistant, supervisor, and then manager, she was responsible for mechanizing financial reporting at a time when personal computers were first seeing widespread use. She earned an M.B.A. at Fordham University in 1984.

A former student and faculty member, Karen Smit Veninga (1967), taught for several years at St. Olaf College, then made an abrupt career change in the mid-1980s when asked to come work in Human Resources for the Baptist Hospital Fund—just as it was preparing to close Mounds Park Hospital. "It was one of the most difficult tasks that I have ever had," she said, "telling my old friends and associates about the change." Later, she took the position as director of human resources for the Minnesota State Senate. Karen was awarded the A. O. Larson Distinguished Alumni Award from the University of Sioux Falls. She has also been named in "Who's Who of American Women."

Alice Hoglund McKee (1948) cared for a family of less prominence but no less importance—her own—after they homesteaded twenty-five miles outside of Fairbanks, Alaska, in 1957. Her nursing skills were put to use with her family. "We had no road, no electricity, no running water, and no medical facilities," she wrote. "I became the health provider for my family and the new families who moved into the community. I am truly grateful for the education I received at Mounds-Midway. The background in nutrition, hygiene, and preventive medicine helped me raise six healthy, strong children."

One of the most unusual jobs held by a Mounds-Midway School of Nursing graduate was given to Jeanne Bjorkman (1960). Following Wendell Anderson's election as governor of Minnesota in 1970, he and his wife, Mary, turned to their family physician, Dr. Vernon Sommerdorf for advice on the best way to care for their three children in the face of a busy public schedule. Dr. Sommerdorf delivered all three children at Mounds Park Hospital, where the Andersons were greatly impressed by the warm, friendly concern of the competent nurses who cared for their babies and for Mrs. Anderson. The doctor recommended Jeanne, who had gained a reputation as one of Mounds Park Hospital's best pediatric nurses after five years of service in that department. Joined by her roommate, Karen Faugust (1962), also a Mounds-Midway graduate, she moved into the carriage house apartment in back of the Governor's Mansion on Summit Avenue. She continued to work with the Anderson family for several years.

The school has proved a fertile ground for authors.

Joyce Buhler Penner (1963) is probably the best-selling former Mounds-Midway graduate. An internationally-recognized sexual therapist, educator and speaker, she and her husband, Cliff, have together written eight books, including *Men and Sex* (winner of the Christian Booksellers Association Gold Medallion), *52 Ways to Have Fun, Fantastic Sex*, and *What Every Woman Wants Her Husband to Know About Sex*. Following her years in Saint Paul, she pursued a B.S. in nursing from the University of Washington, followed by a master's degree in psychosomatic nursing and nursing education from UCLA. She has appeared on *Focus on the Family* and other popular Christian media.

When Nurses Christian Fellowship began publishing the *Journal of Christian Nursing*, they asked Marilyne Backlund Gustafson (1954) to participate on their review panel. As an author, she has contributed to several Nurses Christian Fellowship publications and at seminars to teach spiritual care here and at international conferences. And, suggesting the breadth of talent found among MMSN graduates, she has a ministry with clowning.

Others wrote about their missionary experiences. Annabell Christopherson Weber (1943) wrote *My Cup Runneth Over*, an account of missionary service with Wycliffe Bible Translators in Peru and Columbia, where she worked with her husband, Don. Annabell died in 1999. Grace Thiebold McGill (1947) wrote *The Path of Life* (Belleville: Guardian Books, 2001). The book relates her work in bringing a language to literacy among the Tayal, a tribal group. Woven into the translation projects is the story of their family, based on missionary prayer letters and her husband's notes.

After working in private practice for thirty-eight years, Gladys Thorson Newman (1940) wrote two novels. The subject of one book, *Natalie*, was a semi-autobiographical story about a young woman who attends Mounds-Midway School of Nursing.

Bonnie Erichsen Scherer (1962) turned her writing talents toward children's books, including such charming tales as *The Rescue of Rusty Rabbit* and *Benny's New Home*.

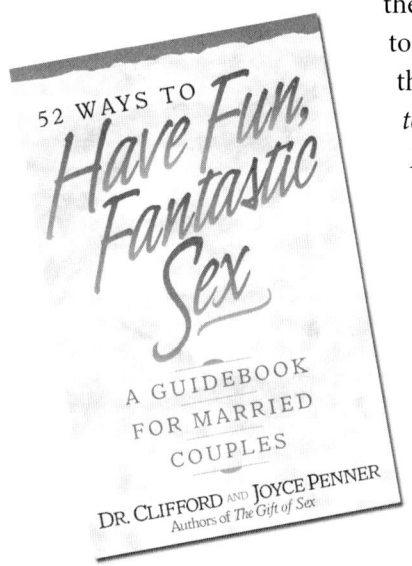

The author, Joyce Buhler Penner (1963) is a highly-sought-after consultant.

No summary of the life and experiences of the graduates of Mounds-Midway would be really accurate without a nod to the majority of alumni who never won a major award, never earned a doctorate, and never wrote a book. They were not military heroes or missionaries — they took nursing jobs where they could and built their lives around the demands of family.

Here is one story, one life. Mildred Willeke was born on December 11, 1909, in the home built by her father in 1904 on Nash Street, Aplington, Iowa, and she lived there much of her life. She graduated from Mounds-Midway in 1931, then worked in St. Paul, Minneapolis and, during World War II, in the Des Moines Munitions Plant. After her brother, Howard, was killed in the invasion of Guam on July 21, 1944, she returned to Aplington to care for her aging parents.

Mildred served for many years as the school nurse for the Aplington, Parkersburg and New Hartford Public Schools, and was a familiar figure for decades of Butler County school children. At the Aplington Baptist Church, she served as a Sunday School teacher, church clerk, co-leader of the Girls' Guild and Baptist Youth Fellowship, and choir member.

A devoted Christian, her obituary said that her knowledge of the Bible, achieved through many decades of careful study, was legendary. She generously supported the mission work of the North American Baptist General Conference, and, when Laura Reddig came back on furlough, graciously lent her car to her friend so that Laura could learn how to drive, practicing her parallel parking out in a back pasture.

When Mildred died in 2003, her six nieces and nephews and six great-nieces and nephews fondly remembered being cared for through many illnesses by "Aunt Mildred, our nurse." One wrote that, for them, "the touch of her skilled hand on a fevered forehead was the beginning of healing."

Alumni Association

Ever since 1909, the Alumni Association has carried on the work of bringing the school's graduates together for service to others, for sharing of life stories, and, of course, for a little fun. It is an important professional association, where graduate nurses can meet together, discuss current trends in nursing and in medicine, and maintain contacts with other graduates through the newsletter and annual meetings.

The purpose of the association, as stated in 1991, has been:

The Class Reunion

Since its inception, the Alumni Association has encouraged graduates to get together with former classmates on important anniversaries.

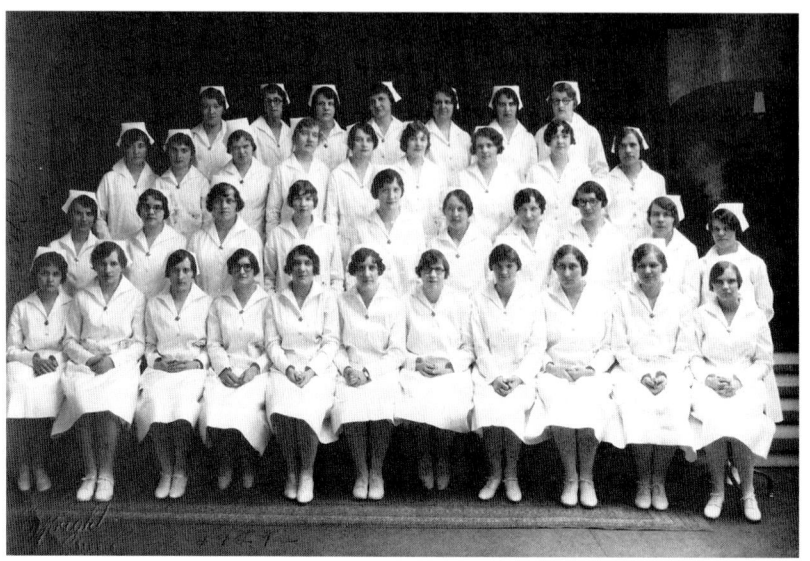

Class of 1929. Bottom: Edith Wilson, Myrtle Melby, Irene Samuelson, Ruth Toussaint, Laura Larson, Lucille Crane, Hazel Anderson, Agnes Bragda, Edith May, Viola Shalgren, Astrid Larson. 2nd R: Ruth Carlson, Dorothy Lundin, Florence Jacobson, Velma Klien, Irene Daleen, May Carlson, Helen Lampie, Ruby Anderson, Anna Lunak. 3rd R: Alice Johnson, Claudia Irish, Keo Kessler, Jennie Nelson, Edna Pearson, Lillian Benson, Ellen Engstrom, Amanda Blumhagen, Mathilda Flood. 4th R: Miriam Dallmus, Ethel Swanson, Evelyn Juenke, Caroline Krueger, Irene Schieslad, Evelyn Peterson, Ruth Dallmus

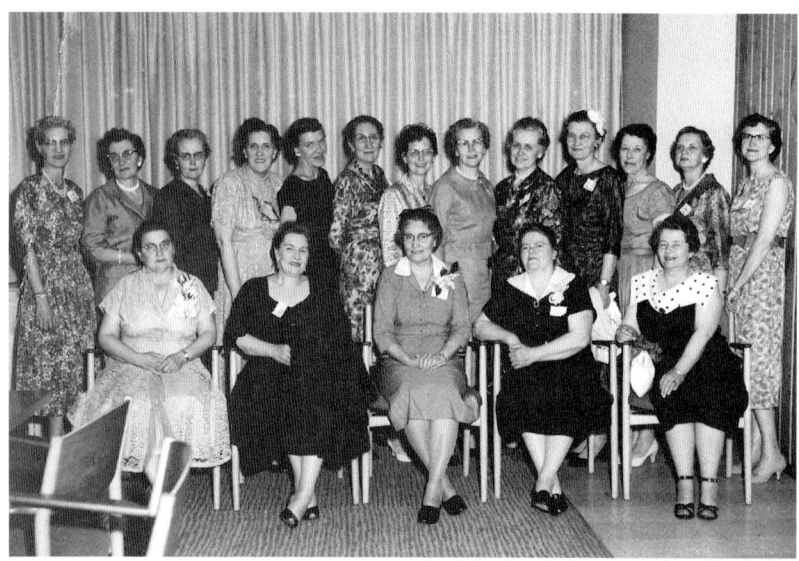

Class of 1929, 1959 reunion. Top: Agnes Bragdon McGuire, Alice Johnson Youngquist, Edith Wilson Ourkey, Lucille Crane Reimers, Laura Larson, Edith May, Ruth Carlson Beck, Ethel Swanson Gunderson, Irene Schiebstad Smyth, Viola Shalgren Larson, Evelyn Juneke Cathcart, Astrid Larson DeVries, Ruth Toussaint Kilbe. Bottom: Claudia Irish Erickson, Lillian Benson Peters, Myrtle Carlson, Anne Lunak Dvaorak, Ellen Engstrom

- To promote interest, friendship, and camaraderie through the annual meeting and luncheon.
- To promote nursing education by maintaining our scholarship fund and by awarding scholarships.
- To preserve our nursing heritage.
- To provide assistance to students.

The annual meetings continue to provide an occasion for graduates to spend a day together, reminisce about school days, and catch up on the latest news.

In 2000, the Alumni Association sponsored a tour to London, where participants visited sites associated with Florence Nightingale. Shirley Streif Christenson (1952) said, "I remember fifty years ago learning about Florence Nightingale, but it seemed old and dry and uninteresting until I got to London." It proved to be a joyous time of learning and friendship. Marilyne Backlund Gustafson described one special day, "It is difficult to decide which site was most meaningful, but our visit to Florence Nightingale's grave outside St. Margaret's thirteenth century church in West Wellow was one of them. It was raining when we drove through the lush English countryside to the cemetery, but the skies cleared and the sun shone as we placed red roses on her grave." [13]

Preserving a common heritage plays a significant role for the Alumni Association. Ruth Gustafson, who served on the faculty for nearly forty years, preserved artifacts from Mounds Park Hospital and early School of Nursing years and displayed them in rooms in Robert Earl Hall. When Mounds Park Hospital closed, these items were transferred to the Midway Dormitory and placed in storage.

In 1991 HealthEast Midway offered the alumni space for a historical museum on 5 North and the board accepted. Mary Jo Borglund Monson was asked to organize a historical society board of directors. The stored artifacts, plus other donations from Midway Hospital and individuals, were moved into the new space and put on display in the museum. In 1993, that group was recognized by the State of Minnesota as a non-profit corporation. When Midway Hospital closed in 1997, HealthEast offered another space on 3 North, further encouraging their efforts to collect additional artifacts, photographs, and documents. In 2003, HealthEast offered a space of 1,300 square feet on the main floor in the corporate tower where it is now located. This further encouraged the Association to carry out its mission: "To collect and preserve the historical knowledge of our nursing heritage for educational, scientific, and social purposes."

The Alumni Association, though, is not just about the past. Its scholarship program offers graduates the opportunity to further their education. In addition, when Mounds-Midway closed, its endowment funds, amounting to $200,000, were transferred to Bethel College for the purpose of "educating Christian nurses." Each year, Bethel University awards five $1000 scholarships to incoming freshmen, renewed as long as the student remains in the nursing program.

Only a few years after the school closed, the Baptist Hospital Fund merged with several other medical organizations to form HealthEast. Soon after, Mounds Park Hospital shut its doors. Then, in 1997, Midway Hospital closed and was converted to an outpatient center. The dorm at 425 Aldine was torn down to make way for a parking lot. But some things remain.

On the day that Mary Danielson was laid to rest, at the funeral service, the congregation sang a few of her favorite hymns, including *Great is Thy Faithfulness* and *Day by Day*. Then, at the request of the nurses from Mounds Park, they closed with *Blest Be the Tie that Binds*, the song that was sung on each student's last day on the floor before graduation.

It has been twenty-four years since the last graduating class and some of the strongest links to the past are no longer with us. What remains is the "fellowship of kindred minds"—women, and a few men, who were called to serve others—to offer the "beginning of healing" with knowledge, skill, and compassion.

Blest be the tie that binds
Our hearts in Christian love;
The fellowship of kindred minds
Is like to that above.

Endnotes

[1] Mary Ann Seawall, "She Nurses Patients' Grudge," *Washington Post*, 25 December 1967.

[2] Sister Helen Kyllingstad's story is included in Carolyn H. Smeltzer and Frances R. Vlasses, *Ordinary People, Extraordinary Lives: The Stories of Nurses* (Indianapolis, IN: Sigma Theta Tau International, 2003).

[3] *Mounds-Midway News Letter*, 13 (December 1948), 13.

[4] See Marilyne Gustafson, "Prayer," in M. Snyder, *Independent Nursing Interventions* (Albany, NY: Delmar Publishing, Inc., 1992), 280-286. Elizabeth A. Peterson, " The Physical, the Spiritual. Can you meet all of your patient's needs?" *Journal of Gerontological Nursing*, 11(10):23-27.

[5] *Mounds-Midway News Letter*, 7 (April 1945), 5-6.

[6] *Mounds-Midway News Letter*, 7 (April 1945), 7-8.

[7] Obituary, *Minneapolis Star-Tribune*, 8 August 2002.

[8] Kelly Grinsteinner, "The Army's angel in white," *Hibbing Daily Tribune*, 11 November 2005.

[9] *Lake Oswego Review*, 26 February 2004; *The Oregonian*, 9 February 2004.

[10] Ruby Eliason, "Time has told the story," *The Standard*, 85 (July 1995), 9.

[11] John Piper, *Don't Waste Your Life* (Wheaton, IL: Crossway Books, 2003).

[12] *Arkansas Gazette*, 11 August 1946.

[13] *Mounds-Midway Alumni Association Newsletter* (2001), 3.

In Service

Mounds-Midway School Of Nursing
Career Missionaries

Year	Name	Board	Field
1911	Esther Hokanson	ABC	China
1917	Rosalie Olson	BAPT. CH	Alaska/Mexico
1920	Constance Olson		Church-NYC, Mexico
1922	Margaret Rinell Jewett	ABC	China
1923	Edna Michaelson Anderson	ABC	Assam
1924	Elsie Larson	ABC	So India
1925	Ruth Johnson Berg	ABC	Burma
1925	Margaret Lang	SIM	Nigeria
1929	Mae Halstenrud	CBHMB	Arizona
1929	Myrtle Carlson	SIM	Nigeria
1929	Irene Daleen Manassa Erickson	ABC	Burma/Lebanon
1929	Edna Pearson Holm	ABC BGC	Assam
1931	Elna Forsell Avey	ABC	Assam
1931	Almyra Eastland Anderson	ABC	Assam
1934	Laura Reddig	NAB	Cameroon
1936	Violet Nelson	ABC	Nicaragua
1938	Sr. Helen Kjllingstad	BSA	North Dakota
1939	Gwendolyn Spry	ABC	N Mexico/Alaska
1939	Joy Philips	BGC	Assam
1942	Ethel Ahlquist Hagstrom	BGC	Assam
1943	Annabel Christofferson Weber	WBT	Peru/Columbia
1943	Arlene Jensen Callaway	BGC GMU	Assam/Morocco
1943	Elsie Johnson Calhoun	BGC	Ethiopia
1944	Arleone Skiff	GMU	Mali
1944	Beatrice Bennett McKenzie	CBFMS	Africa
1945	Delores Wahl Richmond	WBT	Bolivia/Ecuador Peru
1946	Dorothy Lee Cotto-Thornor	LAM	Costa Rica
1946	Elsie Funk Wessman	BGC	Japan
1946	Constance Lindblom Bjelland	BGC	P.I.
1946	Eleanor Weisenberger	NAB	Cameroon
1947	Grace Theobald Mcgill	PRES. CAN.	Taiwan
1947	Shirley Keieman Boyer	SIM	Nigeria

1947	Betty Hotchkiss Nielsen	EV. LUTH	S. Rhodesia Zuzuland Swaziland
1947	Edna Carlson Hughes	ABC	Iran
		IIM	Pakistan
1948	Elaine Berden Carpenter	SIM	Dahomey
1948	Gwen Ticknor	FAITH	Arkansas
1949	Esther Brygger Kile	CBFMS	Congo Bel. Rawanda Uganda
1949	Ruth Duncomb Kreuther	CBFMS	Congo Bel
1949	Mildred Schultz Bryant	BMM	Chad
1949	Wyla Weekly Griggs	BMM	Congo Bel, So.Africa
1949	Esther Wiens Wood	MEN	Columbia
1949	Grace Seibel Thiessen	MCC	Paraguay
1949	Betty Miller Wilson	SBC	Brazil, Germany
1950	Betty Person	BGC	Assam
1950	Irene Piper Shank	CMA	Gabon/ Chad
1950	Betty June Shakleton	AG	Gold Coast
1950	Elaine Westlund Coleman	BGC	Ethiopia
1951	Gloria Geizler Mosiman	TWR	Ecuador
1951	Ruby Eliason	BGC	Assam Cameroon
1951	Kathryn Sheffler Earl	WBT	Mexico
1952	Evelyn Severe Johnson	WBT	Bolivia
1952	Margaret Parker Hoff	CBFMS	Brazil
1952	Arlene Gerdes Derksen	MEN BRE	Congo Bel
1952	Janis Harris Remington Vasterling	ABC	P. I.
1953	Beverly Fillips Donner	WBT	Vietnam
1953	Barbara Kieper	NAB	Cameroon
1953	Ruth Bertell	BGC	Assam
1954	Carol Mosal Osterhus	MAF,GMU	Ecuador
1954	Ruth Huber Baxter	TWR	Ecuador
1955	Marjorie Siemans Geary	CBFMS	Indonesia
1955	Virginia Carlson Steinkamp	CMA	Vietnam
1956	Mavis Johnson Ogren	BGC	Brazil
1958	Donna Randall Carmen	IND	India
1958	Edna Esther Johnson	ECLA	Liberia
1960	Nancy Sandberg Bulcha	BGC	Ethiopia
1960	Joann Sundberg Wright	BGC	Japan
1961	Ulla Tervonen Smith	WEC	W. Africa
1961	Joy Congdon	WBT	Peru
1964	Carol Radke Kjer	SIM	Liberia
1965	Ruth Erickson Gollings	BGC	Mexico
1966	Karen Okerland Beach	CBI	Hongkong

1967	Carol Erickson Kalmbacher	WBT	Indonesia, P.I.
1969	Diana Stuhr	WBT	P.I.
1970	Rebekah Osell	BGC	Ethiopia
1972	Nancy Beaver James	ABC	Haiti
1972	Yema Museu Lahahi	GBGM	Kenya
1972	Judith Swanson Richardson	BEE	E. Europe
1975	Colleen Dewing Sugimoto	AIM	Kenya/Congo
1975	Jane Vandenberg	CBI	Ivory Coast
1975	Donna Zea Roths	PI	Uzbekistan
1976	Sandra Dennis Torjesen	TEAM	Taiwan, Indonesia, China
1976	Cindy Thompson Charles	NAZ	Rawanda
1981	Margaret Calloway Pearson	SBC	Ethiopia
1983	Jennifer Munger	WBT	Russia/Soviet Union

MISSION BOARDS

ABC	American Baptist Convention
AFBC	Afghan Border Crusade
AG	Assemblies Of God
AIM	Africa Inland Mission
BGC	Baptist General Conference
BSA	Benedictine Sisters Annunciation Monastery
BEE	Bible Education Extension
BM M	Baptist Mid Missions (Garb)
CBFMS/CBI	Conservative Baptist Foreign Missionary Society (World Venture)
CBHMS	Conservative Baptist Home Missionary Society
CMA	Christian Missionary Alliance
CMML	Christian Mission to Many Lands
EV LUTH	Evangelical Lutheran
FAITH	Non-Denominational Faith Mission
GBGM	General Board Of Global Ministries (Methodist)
GMU	Gospel Missionary Union (Avant)
IIM	Iran Interior Mission
IND	Independent
LAM	Latin America Mission
MAF	Missionary Aviation Fellowship
MCC	Mennonite Central Committee
MENN	Mennonite
MEN BRE	Mennonite Bretheran
NAB	North American Baptist
NAZ	Nazarene

PI	People Incorporated
PRES/CAN	Presbyterian Church Of Canada
PSP	People Serving People
SBC	Southern Baptist Convention
SIM	Sudan Interior Mission
TEAM	The Evangelical Alliance Mission
TWR	Trans World Radio
WEC	World Evangelical Crusade International
WBT	Wycliffe Bible Translators

Index

A

Abrahamson, Elsie 95
Adams, Jeanette Mundheim 59
Addington, Hazel Ahlstrom 25, 34
Alfaro, Cordelia Kuhn 86, 87, 89, 94
Allert, Maxine Sigfred 59
Alumni Association iii, iv, 36, 57, 60, 161, 167, 168, 169, 171
Ames, Marilyn Oliver 84
Ancker Hospital 61, 64, 75, 88, 89, 97, 110
Anderson, Almyra Eastlund 28, 57, 58
Anderson, Edna Michaelson 26
Anderson, Eunice 117
Anderson, Hurst R. 78
Anderson, Judith 107, 118
Anderson, Lois D. 111, 140, 148
Anderson, Virginia 124, 127, 133
Asbury School of Nursing 78, 79, 80, 81, 100, 101
Assam, India 26, 28, 57, 58, 102, 175, 176
Austin, Gerry 95
Avey, Elna Forsell 58
Axelson, Jeanne 63

B

Junior-Senior Banquet 53
Baptist Hospital Fund 76, 79, 101, 107, 120, 121, 123, 124, 138, 140, 165, 169
Bauer, Jim 134
Baxter, Ruth Huber 90, 93, 162
Bell, Marion 61
Benson, June Evers 47
Benson, Marilyn Moberg 93
Berg, Marjorie 97, 145
Berg, Ruth Johnson 26
Bergh, Selma 16
Bergstrom, Rose 25
Berlin, Florence Jacobson 42
Bernhardson, Lois 131

Bethel College 3, 5, 6, 11, 12, 13, 76, 77, 81, 107, 111, 123, 127, 138, 139, 140, 149, 169
Bibelheimer, Jeanette 118
Biebighauser, Beverly 88
Bjorkman, Jeanne 165
Bloomquist, Jan 130
Blue Cross 44, 71
Bolton-Bailey Act 60
Bonin, Betty 67
Boomer, Judy Magnuson 111, 117, 119, 121, 123, 145
Brace, Genevieve Sutton 81, 86
Brandt, Kathleen Shaw 115
Breitenfeldt, Betty Wolfangle 90
Brethorst, Dr. Alice 79, 80
Brisley, Sandra Barton 164
Brodt, Dagmar Swanburg 5, 148, 149
Brown, Esther Voetmann 146
Brown Report 75
Bryant, Mildred Schultz 66
Buchan, Valerie 82, 92, 154
Buelow, Susan Sargeant 115
Burns, Dr. Robert 22, 65
Burnside (dormitory) 54, 55, 67
Butkowski, Allen 134

C

Cadet Nurse Corps 60, 61
Cady, Judith Hellquist 145
Callaway, Arlene Jensen 160
Calvin, Arthur 42, 44
Carlson, Bill 67
Carlson, Karen 101
Carlson, Myrtle 58
Case, Bev Desens 135
Children's Hospital 10, 36, 49, 64, 67, 128
Choir 96, 99, 115, 116, 135
Clark, Gladys Kent 146
Cobb Hospital 30, 31, 39

Cohelan, Evelyn Ellis 5, 147, 148
Coleman, Elaine Westlund 98, 161
Conley, L. Melvin 1, 41, 76, 79, 100, 101, 107, 121, 124, 133, 138, 139, 140
Cook, Helen 59
Cranmer, Erla 58
Crocker, Joanne Danielson 84

D

Dadukian, Kathryn Linn 164
Dahl, Barbara Carlson 87
Dahl, Rachel 29
Dahlberg, Rev. E. T. 57
Dahlby, Anna 27, 28
Dahlby, Carl P. 11
Dalton, Fay 90
Danielson, Harriet Peterson 84
Danielson, Mary 18, 25, 29, 34, 35, 42, 43, 45, 48, 53, 58, 60, 71, 76, 79, 101, 102, 123, 170
Davies, James 116, 117, 135, 136, 140
Dean, Sandra Mudder 144
Denner, Ardis Williamson 47, 48, 59, 61
Derkson, Mabel 68, 72
Dexter, Jan Heida 115
Dietrich, Cheryl McBride 110, 131, 136, 137
Dobbertin, Mary 95
Doebbeling, Betty Stahl 155
Donner, Beverly Fillips 162
Dreyer, Connie 129, 131
Drinane, Helen 28
DuCharme, Alys 132
Dumeny, Magda Cadet 108

E

Earl, Dr. George 19, 22, 36, 39, 57, 75, 76, 79, 107, 123
Earl, Dr. John 91
Earl, Dr. Robert 10, 11, 12, 14, 22, 36, 41, 64, 71
Eddy, Donna Larson 59, 67, 69
Edman, Eleanor 139
Edminister, Carol Ann 118

Edwards, Dr. Laura 161
Edwards, Margaret 152
Eliason, Lilyan Renaud 116, 117, 136
Eliason, Ruby 5, 160, 161, 162, 171
Erdmann, Char 88
Ericcson, Irene Menassa 144
Erickson, Anita Smith 117
Erickson, Esther 35
Espelien, Adella Bennett 1, 3, 5, 36, 72, 83, 97, 102, 107, 109, 114, 120, 123, 124, 140, 143, 145
Ewald, Orva 67

F

Fast, Della Hildahl 85
Faugust, Karen 165
Felland, Arlene Lick 4
First Swedish Baptist Church 9
Fischbach, Mary 133
Forsyth, Florence 58
Fortune, Margaret 18, 34
Friedsburg, Ann 34, 35, 41, 79
Fritz, Dorothy Kampher 68

G

Gagstetter, Phyllis 49
Garbisch, Anna 58
Garnett, Esther 87
Gilbert, Virginia (Ginger) 85
Gillette, Arthur 10
Gillette Hospital 49
Glee Club 55, 56, 72
Gong, The 36, 53
Gordh, Arvid 11, 12
Grandin, Annette 47, 70, 76, 80, 118
Groff, Sue Ohmann 116
Grooms, Helen Sammons 49, 51, 53, 55, 62
Grotey, Ardis 61
Guderian, Mary 58
Guest, Maude 32
Gustafson, Lenny 128

Gustafson, Marilyne Backlund 3, 4, 149, 166, 169
Gustafson, Ruth 3, 33, 43, 48, 51, 53, 63, 80, 98, 102, 121, 142, 169

H
Halvorsen, Emily 126, 127, 130
Hamilton, Kathleen McNaughton 153
Hamline University 55, 77, 78, 79, 80, 81, 82, 83, 84, 97, 99, 100, 101, 103, 107, 109, 110
Hammargren, Edith 87
Hammes, Dr. E. 65
Hansen, Karen 138
Harms, Carol Harrison 111, 112, 114, 127, 133, 138
Harris, Jan 95
Harrison, Carol Hart Brown 112
Hemmes, Thelma 85, 86, 87, 162
Hillis, Jeanne 58
Hoffpauir, Myrtle Anderson 93
Hokanson, Esther 26
Holm, Edna Pearson 39, 58
Holsten, Iona Stone 4, 92, 146, 147
Hudek, Muriel Severson 142
Hudson, Katherine Stockfleth 29
Hughes, Edna Carlson 64
Husson, Elizabeth 58

I
Industrial Nursing 109
Isaacson, Ida C. L. 3, 16. 34

J
Jaeger, John 55, 56, 70, 96, 99, 117
Jameson, Helen 144
Jefson, Lois 130
Jessup, Beverly Wall 94
Jewett, Margaret Rinell 26
Johnson, Amy 47
Johnson, Curtis 125, 127, 130
Johnson, Janice Jackson 98, 144
Johnson, Selma 58

Just, Jennie Larsen 88, 95

K
Kalmbacher, Carol Erickson 118
Kampher, Charles 68
Karhu, Gladys Benson 130, 131
Kejr, Carol Radke 115
Kieper, Barbara 158
Kirbach, Esther 28
Kirbach-Dahlby Scholarship 28
Kirsten, Lucille 87, 98
Klippenstein, Carol 112
Kroll, Ivy 4
Kronholm, Eunice Peterson 137
Krueger, Caroline 47, 56
Kruschke, Barb Drier 84
Kuehn, Candyce 143
Kuehn, Gladys George 144
Kuhl, Jeanette 78
Kvitrud, Dr. Gilbert 65
Kyllingstad, Sister Helen 144, 171

L
Lang, Margaret 58
LaPanta, Bonnie 133
Larson, Anna Carlson 25
Larson, Eva Ostergren 65
Larson, Janet Valine 67, 70, 96
Larson, Magnus 11, 12, 13
Larson, Marilyn 95
Larson, Olivia Geidd 142
Ledeboer, Vonna Shearer 90
Lee, Dorothy 113, 114, 115, 133, 137
Leitch, Dr. Archibald 65
Lemon, Bernice Thorson 42, 49, 61
Lennberg, Virginia 66
Lick, Arlene 98
Lilja, Lorraine 126, 127, 130
Lindahl, Nels 9, 12, 13
Lindahl, Rachel Ostrom 82, 93

Index

Luhahi, Yema Museu 158
Lumsden, Margaret 59
Lundquist, Carl 107

M
Malmberg, Mrs. 93
Manehr, Emma 58
Manor House (dormitory) 78, 81
Mantzke, Bob 95, 96
Martin, Delores 126
Martin, Ruth 18, 30, 34
May, Lillian Bloom 91, 108
McCrory, Judy Webster 117, 120
McGill, Grace Thiebold 166
McKee, Alice Hoglund 70, 165
McKenzie, Agnes Weins 146
Mears, Norman 107
Merriam Park Hospital 30, 31, 35
Miller, Valerie 133
Miller, Dagney 58
Miller, Jean 124
Miller, Lois 59
Miller, Sheri Gilquist 133
Moberg, Jo Ann Lewis 96
Monk, Caroline 14, 16, 18, 34
Monson, Mary Jo Borglund 4, 83, 89, 92, 169
Moor, Marjorie Sundin 56
Moose Lake State Hospital 111
Mrs. Chase 69, 94, 115
Muchlow, Joanne 114
Myhre, Pearl Jackson 25, 145

N
National League of Nursing 32, 45, 51, 76, 108
Nelson, Violet 28, 47, 48, 69, 82, 83, 84, 98, 102, 142
Newman, Gladys Thorson 49, 71, 166
Nightingale, Florence 53, 84, 169
Northwestern Baptist Hospital Association 30, 39, 42, 44, 71, 75, 76, 101
Nurses' Christian Fellowship 98, 121

Nursing Schools — Today and Tomorrow 45

O
Olan, Ruth 59
Olson, Alice 47
Olson, Charlotte Sandin 91, 127, 133, 134, 139
Olson, Florence 129
Olson, Mary Jenkins 70
Olson, Rosalie 58
Opp, Myrna Kern 119
Ostergren, Edward W. 65
Ostergrew, Effie 43

P
Paquette, Jennie Teberg 16, 17, 36
Parker, Carol 128
Paul, Viola Olson 20, 22
Pearson, Stella Samuelson 70
Pegors, Marie 66
Penner, Joyce Buhler 165
Perron, Clifford 124
Perry's 55, 66, 95
Person, Betty 160
Peter, Judy Kempton 121
Peterson, Elizabeth 5, 127, 128, 133, 149, 171
Peterson, Leona 23

Q
Quamen, Myrtle Nereson 58, 59, 152

R
Radmann, Margaret Edwards 151
Rankin, Dawn Opseth 144
Reddig, Laura 5, 58, 156, 157, 158, 167, 175
Red Cross 27, 28, 49, 59, 146, 149, 164
Reed, Lucille Walter 49
Rich, Faith 116
Riedell, Gracia 89, 91, 97, 100
Riggs, C. Eugene 10, 11, 13, 14, 22, 34, 36
Robertson, Helene Stewart 150, 151

Robertson, Lauralie Nelson 68, 88, 93
Robert Earl Hall 4, 62, 66, 142, 169
Rolfe, Daphne A. 80, 81, 101
Roth, Janice 128
Ruberto-Krugman, Pam 130
Runningen, Lylah 67
Rural Nursing 103, 112
Ryden, Alma 34
Ryden, Karen 28

S
Sandve, Wanyce C. 103, 107, 109, 115, 118, 119, 123, 139, 140
Sanitarium, Battle Creek 11
Scherer, Bonnie Erichsen 109, 115, 117, 166
Schoch, Anne 114
Schottmuller, Gena Testa 1, 2, 85, 90, 92, 96, 145
Schreiber, Marilyn Olson 133
Schwabauer, Arlys Deckert 107, 111, 112, 115, 119
Severe, Evelyn 95
Severson, Muriel 98
Sidlo, Agnes 90
Siebel, Grace 66
Siemans, Margery 88
Sioux Falls College 124, 157, 165
Smith, Gordon 121, 123
Smith, Irene 42, 57
Smith, Naomi 132
Soderberg, Dorothy 49
Sommerdorf, Dr. Vernon 67, 165
Stahnke, Emma Gutsch 54
Stegmeier, Judy 130
Stenstrom, Alice 68, 72
Stevenson, Eula Marienau 82
Stewart, Isabel Maitland 28
Stok, Bobbie 97
Stolp, Joan Carlson 82, 95
Stone, Chester 124
Sugimoto, Colleen Dewing 133
Swackhammer, Violet Isaacson 151

Swanson, Bernice Franck 47
Swenamson, Stephanie Werner 18, 24
Swenson, Olof 11, 12

T
Tervonen, Ulla 118
Tezpur, India 102, 160, 161
Thornquist, Edith 34
Ticknor, Gwendolyn 42, 163
Tofte, Birgit 89
Tolbert, Nora 34
Treleaven, Donna 66
Trost, Stephen 134, 138
Turk, Alice 145

V
Veninga, Karen Smit 115, 124, 165
Vigen, Jolyn Conrad 89, 101, 109
Vogel, Eleanore Anderson 4, 88, 95, 149

W
Wachter, Janet Chatfield 116
Waldron, Diana 114
Waldt, Jean Crandall 97
Wallin, June Anderson 61, 70
Ward, Dr. Peter 44
Warner, Jennie 18
Warnert, Brother Joseph 129, 131
Weber, Annabell Christopherson 166
Whirley, Susanne 143
White, Mary 58
Wilford, Sharon 114
Willeke, Mildred 166
Willie, Paula 115, 131, 132, 135
Wilson, Betty Miller 66
Windham, Carol 126, 130
Wood, Horace 95
World War II 58, 67, 109, 146, 150, 152, 153, 157, 167
Worm, Fern 109
Wright, Joanne 101

Y
Yard, Kris Swanson 134, 135
Yokie, Doris 80
Youngdahl, Bessie 61

Z
Ziehlke, Kurt 139, 156